Overcoming Insurmountable Odds

Overcoming Insurmountable Odds

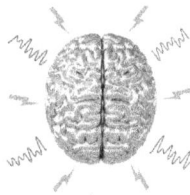

How I Rewired My Brain to Do the Impossible

Scott A. McCreight

The following information is intended for general information purposes only. Individuals should always confer with their healthcare provider before administering any health and athletic protocols or suggestions made in this book. Any application of information set forth in the following pages is at the reader's discretion and is his or her sole responsibility.

"Another in the Fire" by Hillsong United is quoted with licensed permission by Capital CMG Publishing.

For more information about *Overcoming Insurmountable Odds*, or programs listed within, Scott can be reached at Scott@McCreightOnline.net or visit https://www.oioBook.com.

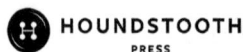

HOUNDSTOOTH PRESS

OVERCOMING INSURMOUNTABLE ODDS
How I Rewired My Brain to Do the Impossible

ISBN	978-1-5445-3551-7	*Hardcover*
	978-1-5445-3550-0	*Paperback*
	978-1-5445-3549-4	*Ebook*

An audiobook version is also available.

Contents

*This book is dedicated to all who have been told,
"No, you can't do that."*

To Betty Taliaferro McCreight—my mom—my greatest advocate.

From even before my birth, you have been there for me. Raising a child with cerebral palsy is never easy for any parent. You fought harder than anyone. Not only did you ensure that I received the very best medical treatments and physical therapies available for my development, but you also tirelessly performed the heavy lifting along my path. From attending countless doctors' meetings, to fighting insurance companies, to watching every PT session I had at the Austin CP Center, you were there. From my unique educational development plan to researching the best CP treatment protocols available, you drove a very dedicated pursuit, educating people along the way, including your son, me. How do you tell your own child he is adopted and he has CP? You have truly been a gift from above. It was never easy for you, but it was very rewarding to those you have ultimately touched along the way. Thanks, Mom.

Faith is powerful.

Faith can move mountains.

"*The human body is truly a miracle in motion—trillions of cells all working together to produce life from matter. Every second, the human body transmits over 100,000 messages that control everything from the heart to the movement of a little toe. These messages (nerve impulses) can travel up to 325 miles per hour across over 45 miles of nerves. Yet, these same nerve impulses can be blocked by pressures that amount to less than the weight of a dime!*"

—DR. GARY SCHREIBER[1]

"*Neuroplasticity[:] the capacity of the brain to develop and change throughout life, something Western science once thought impossible.*"

—ANDREW WEIL, MD[2]

Preface

I HAVE WRITTEN THIS BOOK ENTIRELY FROM MY OWN PERSONAL experiences, memories of places, events, people, research, and conversations with medical and scientific professionals, with supporting data added to explain and educate you, the reader, along the way. Although not word-for-word reenactments, this is every bit the story of my life growing up with a neurological disorder known as cerebral palsy (CP). Others may have a different slant on events that happened over these years, but these are mine. I have changed several names of individuals and organizations to respect their privacy or protect their identities.

My hope for readers is that you will have a richer understanding of what it is like growing up and living with cerebral palsy and how those with CP can transform their lives just as I have. This transformation is not limited to those with CP; it is open to all who want to reach for the sky and move mountains.

May my experiences and research into CP and what it takes to transform one's life spark an even greater lifelong transformation in you.

After consulting many medical definitions over the years, I've come up with my own, which I'd like to share as a beginning point for this journey:

Neuroplasticity—*The brain's inherent ability to rewire itself by forming new neural networks throughout life. Neuroplasticity allows the neurons, also called nerve cells, in the brain to compensate for injury and to adjust their activities in response to new and novel situations.*

Introduction

An old friend of mine once told me, "Scott, you don't seem to do 'easy' very well. But you go straight to 'hard' and master that darn well. Your determination to overcome the 'hard' in life is what truly makes you unique." This statement encapsulates a lot of what this book is about. I was born premature, underweight, and with a neurological condition called cerebral palsy. From a young age, I was sent a clear message: any number of activities should have been easy, and I should have been able to do them. But for whatever reason, my body didn't get that message, and those activities weren't easy. Some even said they were impossible.

Instead of letting it dictate my life, I obliterated that message to overcome and triumph. I refused to play by *those rules*. Rather than focus on simple activities, I skipped right over them and went to the very things that others found difficult, and I showed them (and perhaps proved to myself) what I was really capable of.

Maybe you also have CP, or you have a friend or loved one who does. Perhaps you are a physical therapist or a personal trainer wanting to "raise the bar" with your clients, to build their self-confidence and uncover abilities they never thought they had, just like I once thought of myself. Or maybe you just like a good story about overcoming overwhelming, insurmountable odds.

Who would have expected that a small, shy, skinny boy with CP would later turn into an engineer, technical scuba instructor, author, skier, athlete, and bodybuilder? I certainly had a lot of doubters along the way, including some of my own therapists and doctors. It hasn't come easily, either. No. As you'll read, I've had more than my fair share of setbacks. But hope, staying positive, sheer motivation, and a determination to excel are the prerequisites to overcome insurmountable odds and achieve unexpected greatness.

In the course of my life and in digging deep to write this book, I've discovered a treasure trove of novel, unique, and innovative methods and techniques to overcome both real and preconceived barriers. Neuroplasticity is a developing concept that you will read about in the following pages. Neuroplasticity is loosely defined as the brain's inherent ability to rewire itself by forming new neural networks throughout life. Neuroplasticity allows the neurons in the brain to compensate for injury and to adjust their activities in response to new and novel situations. I'm not saying I have found the answers or a cure for CP or that these techniques will work for everyone. But they have worked for me as well as many others whom I write about in the pages that follow. Enormously so. As such, I readily share what I have learned in hopes that this will motivate, inspire, and help others.

As my trainers helped me to break barriers and reach new heights, they told me they were willing to pursue new goals with me because of my "raw determination and unbreakable spirit." That's what it takes to overcome difficulties in this life. Some of these difficulties almost broke my spirit, as I will reveal in the pages to come.

Friends of mine even began to think that maybe this neuroplasticity thing I had been talking about really did work. I became a model of proof for these theories. It was no longer just something I had been reading about, studying about, or talking about. I began to live out my own true success story in the making. Perhaps more importantly, several people who had kids with CP or had CP themselves asked how they, too, could benefit from what they saw in me and this transformation.

Along the way, I've adopted this motto: "Cerebral palsy should not keep one from reaching the impossible." And I've deeply internalized Philippians 4:13, for "I can do all things through Christ who gives me strength."

This book will take you on a fantastic journey. I'll give you some background information so we can start on the same page about cerebral palsy. Then I'll start at the beginning of my life as a small, shy boy with CP growing up in a competition water-skiing family. I'll show you how I had to find faith and had to lean on Him even more when complacency sunk in. Finally, you'll travel with me on a roller-coaster ride of new beginnings, transformations, and numerous setbacks, including one so severe I call it "the reckoning." You'll see neuroplasticity in action throughout my entire life, but especially in the times when I specifically pursued it to become an athlete and bodybuilder, in what I call my "transformation." So get ready, for the impossible is about to become possible, and overcoming insurmountable odds is just around the corner.

PART 1

Background

He Never Makes Mistakes

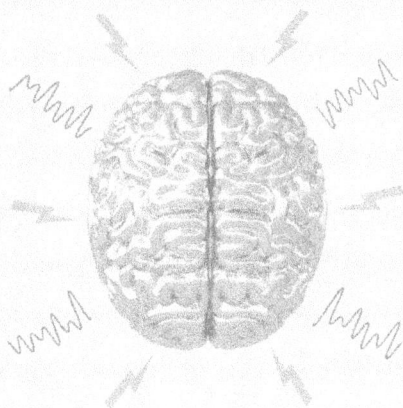

Debunking Myths Surrounding Cerebral Palsy

You might be intimately familiar with CP, or not even know what CP is. If you are "experienced," you might even be tempted to skip this part. I have CP and consider myself a CP "expert." However, I have come to learn some interesting and informative facts about the very condition that affects my everyday life. I encourage you, my reader, to press on through "Debunking Myths Surrounding Cerebral Palsy." You might just learn something new, like I have.

Before we get to my story and what it was like growing up with (and overcoming) cerebral palsy, my desire is to educate you about what *is* and *is not* CP. To debunk so-called common beliefs about CP. Trust me; I have heard it all. In fact, I even believed some of these myths myself. So let's get on the same page regarding CP.

Sadly, many myths about cerebral palsy persist today despite enormous advancements in medical science and research. These myths also produce and propagate stress on families with children or adults who have CP. Unfortunately, during my birth and childhood, people knew even less about CP than they know today. I have to admit, before researching and writing this book, I was unaware there were different types of cerebral palsy; I just knew I had CP.

Cerebral palsy is not hereditary and cannot be passed down by DNA. It is a neuromuscular condition that can affect movement, coordination, speech, and hearing.

The Cerebral Palsy Group—a team of world-class doctors and healthcare professionals dedicated to providing high-quality, medically reviewed data on everything related to cerebral palsy as well as birth-injury topics—has produced a list of seventeen of the most pervasive myths about cerebral palsy and medical answers that dispel these myths.[3] Along with this list I have included clinical information that is helpful for understanding this condition known as CP.

MYTH #1: CP IS A PROGRESSIVE CONDITION

This misconception may come from confusing CP with certain degenerative neurological disorders, such as Tay–Sachs disease and multiple sclerosis. These disorders can worsen as the patient gets older. In contrast, cerebral palsy symptoms do not generally increase in severity and instead may actually improve over time, especially with aggressive physical therapy and exercise. I have found through my own transformation, as well as those that are mentioned in this book, that the more active we are, the less CP affects our overall health. As it turns out, this is true for all of us, whether we have neurological abnormalities or not—the more active we are, the less degradation our bodies experience.

Continued research into surgical and nonsurgical options and other therapeutic strategies have made the latter scenario more common in recent years (the more active we are, the less CP affects our overall health). The key is starting these intensive strategies[4] as soon as possible for longer-lasting benefits. However, even applied later in life, these can, and do, have a transformative affect in people, just like in me.

MYTH #2: PEOPLE WITH CP CAN'T LIVE INDEPENDENTLY

Some people with cerebral palsy may need family and caregiver support throughout their entire lives. However, many adults with CP can be fully independent. Adults with CP who live independently may make use of the following strategies:

- Assistive technologies, including mobility aids and transfer equipment

- Modifications to the home and workplace, such as lower countertops for wheelchair users

- Personal care assistance for potentially difficult tasks, such as household chores

MYTH #3: CHILDREN WITH CP CAN'T COMMUNICATE

While children with cerebral palsy are more likely to also have language disorders and hearing impairments, many do not. Those who do have these challenges may overcome them through speech therapy and the use of alternative communication devices, such as speech boards and computers, to name a few. Technology has gifted the ability to communicate to those who once had no way of communicating before.[5] Tomorrow looks more promising, as technology advancements will make it even easier.

MYTH #4: CHILDREN WITH CP ARE INTELLECTUALLY DISABLED

It is important to remember that while CP is a neurological disorder, it is fundamentally a problem with motor function. Although as many as half of the children with CP also have some level of cognitive impairment, this is not directly related to having CP. Cognitive impairments can range from very mild to severe intellectual disabilities. Children with CP are also more likely than the general population to have learning disabilities—which are distinct from intellectual disabilities and, again, not directly related to CP.

MYTH #5: CP IS THE SAME FOR EVERYONE

Cerebral palsy is actually a broad umbrella term for a diverse group of motor functional neurological disorders that often involve very different symptoms.

The four main types of CP are as follows:

- Spastic cerebral palsy (pyramidal)

- Athetoid cerebral palsy (extrapyramidal or dyskinetic)

- Ataxic cerebral palsy

- Mixed cerebral palsy

Before I explain the various types of CP above, I must first define what *paresis* and *plegia* refer to.

Paresis is defined as a weakened limb or body part, whereas **plegia/plegic** is defined as a paralyzed limb or body part.

These prefixes can be further broken down into the following nine classifications, where prefixes and root words are combined to yield descriptions of the affected body parts.

When used along with the Gross Motor Function Classification System (described in the next chapter), this provides a detailed description of where and to what extent a person is affected by cerebral palsy:

1. **Monoplegia/monoparesis** only affects one limb. May be a form of hemiplegia/hemiparesis where only one limb is significantly impaired.

2. **Diplegia/diparesis** usually indicates the legs are affected more than the arms. Primarily affects the lower body but can affect upper body only.

3. **Hemiplegia/hemiparesis** means that an arm and a leg on same side of the body are affected.

4. **Paraplegia/paraparesis** only affects the lower half of the body, which includes both legs.

5. **Triplegia/triparesis** affects three limbs of the body. This could be both arms and a leg or both legs and an arm. Or it could refer to one upper and one lower extremity and the face.

6. **Double hemiplegia / double hemiparesis** affects all four limbs, but one side of the body is more affected than the other.

7. **Tetraplegia/tetraparesis** affects all four limbs, but three limbs are more affected than the fourth.

8. **Quadriplegia/quadriparesis** affects all four limbs, usually equally.

9. **Pentaplegia/pentaparesis** indicates that four limbs are affected, with neck and head paralysis often accompanied by eating and breathing complications.

Within each of the above is a wide range of symptoms and severities. For example, one person with spastic CP might have trouble controlling a single leg, while another person with the same condition might have quadriplegia with all four limbs severely affected. A person's specific needs and challenges will be unique to each individual, as no two cases of CP are ever the same. This is one of many mysteries I have uncovered in understanding my own affliction. Although all cases of CP are unique in challenges and needs, proven protocols and treatments can be successfully applied to all.

Keep in mind that the brain injury that causes cerebral palsy affects motor functioning. It influences the ability to control the body in a desired manner and does not generally affect cognitive functioning.

There are two classifications of motor functioning: spastic and non-spastic. Both can have multiple variations, and it is possible to have a mixture of both types.

Spastic cerebral palsy is characterized by increased muscle tone (tight or rigid).

Non-spastic cerebral palsy will exhibit decreased or fluctuating muscle tone (loose or flaccid).

Here is a little bit about **muscle tone**:

Many motor function terms describe cerebral palsy's effect on proper muscle tone and how muscles work together. For example, properly bending an arm is a balanced movement, like a ballet dance. This movement requires the biceps to contract and the triceps to relax together in a precise balance or "dance" so that it is not jerky, spastic, or floppy. When muscle tone is impaired due to CP, muscles tend not to work together and can even work in opposition to one another (spastic).

Muscle tone is defined as follows:

Hypertonia/hypertonic—Increased muscle tone, resulting in very stiff limbs and associated with spastic cerebral palsy.

Hypotonia/hypotonic—Decreased muscle tone, often resulting in loose, floppy limbs and associated with non-spastic cerebral palsy.

MYTH #6: COLLEGES DO NOT ACCOMMODATE STUDENTS WITH CEREBRAL PALSY

It is increasingly common for young adults with cerebral palsy to pursue a college education. In the US, colleges that receive federal funding—the vast majority of institutions of higher education—are legally required to make accommodations for all disabled students, including those with CP. Even many colleges that don't receive federal funding often voluntarily aid students with CP. Accommodations may include following the recommendations outlined in a student's individualized education program as well as ensuring accessibility to campus facilities. Having CP won't prevent people from receiving a quality education. My story of going to college and earning multiple degrees serves as strong testimony that this myth has been debunked.[6]

MYTH #7: CEREBRAL PALSY IS ALWAYS CAUSED BY MEDICAL MALPRACTICE

Cerebral palsy is caused by damage to the brain before, during, or shortly after a child's birth. It could also be due to a condition that results in the brain failing to develop properly. This may be mediated by injury, inflammation, or a lack of oxygen. While it's true that some cases of CP may be caused by medical malpractice, many are not.

Common Causes of CP Include

- Serious maternal infection during pregnancy

- Brain infections after birth, such as meningitis

- Birthing complications, including forceps delivery

- Head trauma (traumatic brain injury)

- Congenital disorders, such as heart defects and issues with blood clotting

- Medication errors

- Maternal substance abuse

Factors That Increase the Risk for CP Include

- Premature birth

- Low birth weight

- Multiple births (e.g., twins or triplets)

- Certain infertility treatments that increase the chance of having multiple births

- Maternal health conditions, such as seizures and thyroid disorders

MYTH #8: PARENTING A CHILD WITH CP IS OVERWHELMING

Raising any child is no easy task, and it's true that it can become even more difficult for parents of children with disabilities. However, CP can vary in severity and therefore requires a varying degree of parental care.

Today, a great deal of support is available to families of those with cerebral palsy. These resources range from monetary help to faith-based support and practical guidance. Simply being able to talk to others who know what you're going through can and often does help as well. This means that while raising a child with CP can be challenging at times, it does not need to be overwhelming, nor does it have to be done alone. This also applies to those affected with CP. Support groups are crucial. Growing up with CP and not talking with others about my struggles made my childhood even more difficult, as I will share further into my story.

MYTH #9: A CHILD WITH CEREBRAL PALSY HAS A LIMITED FUTURE

It's true that people with CP generally have shorter-than-average life expectancies and that some with more severe forms of CP may not make it to adulthood. However, many children with CP end up living long, fulfilling lives. Simply having CP does not prevent a person from developing close friendships, finding romance, or accomplishing great and amazing things, as I will amply demonstrate within this book.

MYTH #10: PEOPLE WITH CP WILL NEVER HAVE CHILDREN OF THEIR OWN

Parents of children with CP may feel disheartened by the possibility of never having grandchildren. The truth is that many adults with CP can and do have children of their own. Cerebral palsy does not generally impact a person's fertility. Additionally, only a minority of CP cases are caused by genetic disorders, and CP is not hereditary—adults with CP do not have to worry about passing the condition down to their children.

Some parents with CP may choose to adopt for medical reasons, while others opt to have biological children. While they may be at greater risk for complications, even women with more severe forms of CP can experience successful pregnancies and give birth to healthy children. Others with the condition may decide maternal surrogacy is a better choice.

MYTH #11: A PERSON WITH CP WILL NEVER HAVE A CAREER

While it's unfortunately true that people with disabilities face higher rates of unemployment, many people with CP do have successful careers. People with CP can be found in almost any field. Successful professionals with CP include actors, scientists, engineers, authors, and even athletes (in my case, all of the last four—I'm still working on the first). Some, such as pediatric neurologist Janice Brunstrom-Hernandez, MD, even go on to help improve the lives of future generations of children with CP.

MYTH #12: CHILDREN WITH CEREBRAL PALSY CAN NEVER LEARN TO WALK

It's true that some children with CP will always need to rely on mobility aids, such as wheelchairs or walkers, to get around. However, this is by no means the norm. In fact, over half of the people with CP do not require mobility aids at all. While they may walk slowly or with a different gait, children with cerebral palsy may indeed learn to walk independently. Additionally, some may have no trouble walking at all, as CP doesn't always affect the lower limbs.

Medical advancements are helping children and adults walk with the implementation of neuroplasticity and through electrical muscle stimulation ("ESM" or "ESTIM") therapy (more on both of these topics later in the book).

MYTH #13: PEOPLE WITH CP WILL ALWAYS HAVE LIMITED MOBILITY

Even those who can't walk aren't necessarily homebound. Assistive technologies can help wheelchair users stay just as active as people who are independent walkers. For example, modifications to motor vehicles can mean that even children who experience paraplegia can learn to drive once they reach their teens. Additionally, more and more communities are investing in accessibility measures, such as curb ramps and wider sidewalks, which help to ensure that people with mobility impairments can freely enjoy the outdoors.

MYTH #14: CEREBRAL PALSY IS UNTREATABLE

For a long time, medical science believed that CP *was* untreatable and that the brain, once damaged, is irreparable (known as the outdated "brain is rigid" concept).[7] However, thanks to research pioneers like Dr. Karen Pape and others, this myth has not been true for decades. Today, children can benefit from a wide variety of cerebral palsy treatments, ranging from intensive physical therapy to medications for co-occurring conditions. Through these therapeutic interventions, parents may see their children's symptoms improve over time, sometimes significantly. Medical advancements are today helping children and adults in the areas of neuroplasticity and ESTIM therapy (more later in this book on both topics).

MYTH #15: CP IS CURABLE

While there are methods of managing CP, there is no current way to cure this condition.

However, that doesn't mean that there will never be a cure for cerebral palsy! The latest research in regenerative medicine and neuroplasticity is quite promising for people living with neurological disorders. Children born with CP today may see a true cure for the disorder within their lifetimes.

MYTH #16: CP IS RARE

Cerebral palsy is the number one childhood motor disability and one of the most common causes of chronic disability in children in general. Cerebral palsy affects as many as 1 in 323 children.[8] If you think you've never known someone with CP, you may be wrong; mild cases often go unnoticed in adults. I'll introduce you to some of these adults later in the book. I have even been asked by medical staff if I am *sure* I have CP.[9]

MYTH #17: THERE ARE NO RESOURCES FOR CHILDREN WITH CP AND THEIR FAMILIES

As previously stated in debunking myth #8, there is a large network of support for parents and caregivers to turn to, including:

- Financial assistance for medical expenses

- Legal counseling for cases of suspected medical malpractice

- College scholarships

- Advice and parenting tips

- Accessibility strategies

Now that we understand what CP is and is *not*, let's discuss more about how CP is classified.

The Gross Motor Function Classification System

WHILE GROWING UP WITH CP IS OFTEN CHALLENGING, IT IS IMPORTANT for those affected to know the realities of our disorder; these realities should not involve limits on who we can be and what we will ultimately be able to accomplish. Likewise, parents of children with CP will indeed encounter hardships, but these challenges are not certain and are often overcome, as I will demonstrate throughout this book.

The Gross Motor Function Classification System (GMFCS) is a measure that describes a person's ability to move throughout daily life. Today, the GMFCS is used by the following groups:

1. Professionals and researchers, to better understand the needs of people with CP and to develop standards of care

2. Therapists, clinicians, and surgeons, to help families understand a child's current abilities, identify what interventions/supports are most appropriate for them, and determine how often a child should be monitored for hip dysplasia and other conditions commonly seen in people with cerebral palsy

3. Parents or persons with CP, to help with understanding the imme-
    diate needs and realistic next steps/goals for you or your child. Once
    you know your or your child's GMFCS, you should take this infor-
    mation to a professional care team to discuss how this affects your
    ongoing care plan.

In a recent survey of parents of children with CP, most caregivers reported
that they preferred to learn about their child's GMFCS level, but less than half
of the survey participants had this information. Eighty-three percent of caregivers said it would be helpful to revisit this information over time.[10]

Beginning in 1997, experts began charting and categorizing the gross motor
function of youngsters with cerebral palsy using the following five levels of
the GMFCS (expanded and revised in 2007 to include an age band for youth
from twelve to eighteen years old). This system is usually applied between the
ages of twelve months and twelve years old.[11] GMFCS distinctions between
levels are generally based on functional abilities, the need for assistive technology, and, to a much lesser extent, quality of movement. It is important to
remember that these five GMFCS levels are only guidelines, and children with
CP may not exactly fit into just one category. After all, cerebral palsy affects
each individual in unique ways, and sometimes we cannot be easily placed
into nice, neat classifications.

The Cerebral Palsy Alliance has created a general representation of the
GMFCS as a guide for basic understanding of motor functioning for kids
between the ages of six and twelve years old.[12]

GMFCS Level I

Children walk at home, at school, outdoors, and in the community.
They can climb stairs without the use of a railing. Children perform

gross motor skills such as running and jumping, but speed, balance, and coordination are limited.

GMFCS Level II

Children walk in most settings and climb stairs holding on to a railing. They may experience difficulty walking long distances and balancing on uneven terrain, on inclines, in crowded areas, or in confined spaces.

Children may walk with physical assistance, such as a handheld mobility device, or use wheeled mobility over long distances. Children have only minimal ability to perform gross motor skills such as running and jumping.

GMFCS Level III

Children walk using a handheld mobility device in most indoor settings. They may climb stairs holding on to a railing with supervision or assistance. Children use wheeled mobility when traveling long distances and may self-propel for shorter distances.

GMFCS Level IV

Children use methods of mobility that require physical assistance or powered mobility in most settings. They may walk for short distances at home with physical assistance or use powered mobility or a body support walker when positioned. At school, outdoors, and in the community, children are transported in a manual wheelchair or use powered mobility.

GMFCS Level V

Children are transported in a manual wheelchair in all settings. Children are limited in their ability to maintain head and trunk postures against the forces of gravity and to control leg and arm movements.

GMFCS level descriptions are copyrighted by Palisano et al. (1997) Dev Med Child Neurol 39:214-23 CanChild, http://www.canchild.ca/

Now that I have discussed the basics of CP and how to classify severity, I want to share where some of my most painful and cherished early memories and treatment took place. A little place in Austin, Texas, called the Austin Cerebral Palsy Center (Austin CP Center).

History of the
Austin CP Center

AFTER I WAS BORN AND MY PARENTS LEARNED THAT I HAD CP,[13] THEY needed a facility where I could receive physical therapy, occupational therapy, care, and family support. My primary care doctor introduced my parents and me to the Austin Cerebral Palsy Center. During my time researching back stories for this book, I discovered the origins of the Austin CP Center and what became of this institution. I found an incredibly rich history of professionals with a desire to bring the very best care to those most in need, kids like me. Without these dedicated folks and the expert care they provided, my story would be quite different today.

ORIGINS

The Texas Society for Crippled Children was formed in 1937 as the Easter Seals of Central Texas. A decade or so later, in the spring of 1948, a small building was dedicated as the Austin Cerebral Palsy Center, serving a small population of Central Texas residents.

My research into the origins of the Austin CP Center led me to Barbara Watt. Barbara and my mom formed a small support group for parents of kids at the Austin CP Center while I was growing up. I developed a bond with Barbara's son Gavin as we played together as tots.

Upon learning of my research for this book, Barbara was excited and wanted Robin Cooper (maiden name Robin Jones) and me to meet. Robin's father was in the Texas legislature in the late 1940s. Her mother, Bess Jones, had a very strong social standing in Austin politics and was comfortable making *requests* of the mayor, with whom she was on a first-name basis. Needless to say, she used these connections to pull some pretty big strings and was able to get the Austin CP Center started and funded.

I, like many other kids around Austin with CP in the 1970s, am extremely grateful to the Austin CP Center and Bess Jones for setting out to develop and offer the very best care for those with CP. Harris Jones (Bess's son) and I share a bond that I had never experienced before Harris's story came to light. We both have CP, and both of our mothers wanted the best possible care for us. I have now come to know that without Harris's legacy, my story of triumph over CP would be quite incomplete.

HARRIS'S LEGACY

I had the pleasure of interviewing Robin Cooper on the cool afternoon of August 29, 2020. We met at Robin's home in West Austin, not too far from where the Austin CP Center used to be located. Robin was surprised that someone was interested in the Austin CP Center or its origins after all these years. We spoke a bit about my intimate connection with the Austin CP Center. I told her I was a former patient there and that I was writing a book on neuroplasticity and my triumph over CP. Robin was overjoyed that her story would be shared after all these years.

Robin's brother, Harris Jones, was born on Columbus Day, 1945. His birth was complicated, and due to the war effort, there were no doctors present at his birth. The nurses tried unsuccessfully to delay his birth until the doctors could arrive. As a result, he developed CP and seizures shortly after. As I soon discovered, Harris's mother, Bess Jones, was the impetus behind the creation of the Austin CP Center in 1948. My rich conversations with Robin Cooper revealed a treasure trove of material from her personal collection and memories of her brother, Harris, and their mom, Bess.

She pulled out a family scrapbook filled with pictures and aged articles. One article in particular not only struck me with intense fascination but was also one of Robin's most cherished pieces in her collection. First published in Austin's local newspaper, the *Austin American-Statesman*, this article—included here in its entirety and which she read to me verbatim—was also printed in the May 1958 edition of the *Alcalde*, the alumni magazine of the University of Texas:

Her Heart Helps Them to Walk[14]

This story should be told at Eastertide because it truly reflects Easter's great hope for little children everywhere. It tells how a young mother literally built a new future for Cerebral Palsy children of Austin through her unwavering faith in the goodness of others. It is the story of Mrs. Herman Jones, the former Bess Harris, BJ, class of '34, who worked long hours with untiring effort and determination to make the founding and development of Austin Cerebral Palsy Center possible.

It was in the spring of 1947 that Bess Jones returned to her home in Austin from long travels across the nation, including Washington, DC, in search of adequate aid for her own small, crippled son. She met five other Austin mothers, who also were seeking specialized care for youngsters whose arms and legs were far from sturdy.

At that time there were only a few recognized specialists versed in treating CP children in Chicago, Washington, New York, Maryland, and Philadelphia. The young mother of our story was determined that, somehow or other, care for the CP child should be brought home to Central Texas.

In that same spring period of 1947, Bess Jones told family and friends that she had learned three necessary approaches to (help) aid crippled children, long called "the forgotten children" by medical men who wanted to help but knew very little, scientifically, that is, about the cerebral palsied.

First of all, Mrs. Jones pointed out, she had learned that a cerebral palsied child's only hope for a future of near normalcy was found in the parents' awareness that he or she can be helped. Such a child most often is possessed of a far higher IQ than the so-called normal child. Then, this intrepid young woman was sure that she had to set up two educational programs for this area. One, so that the general public might learn to understand the person with CP and his/her needs; and two, to develop a concentrated education program for parents so that they might gain the knowledge that their child could and would be helped.

She chartered her work so well that in six short months Austin was busily planning an aid program for these youngsters. In January 1948, Mrs. Jones presented a "plan of operation" that she had carefully worked out with officials of the Travis County Society for Crippled

Children, which had become inactive during World War II. This plan was discussed at a luncheon attended by representatives of child welfare agencies, nurses, and doctors, Junior League, and three Panhellenic groups that had adopted international altruistic programs of aid to the cerebral palsied at their first post-war conventions in June 1947.

At that luncheon meeting, the Crippled Children's Society was reorganized with Mrs. Jones as President and the decision was made that Austin would have a CP Center. Officials of the Texas Society for Crippled Children representing a new CP Center in Dallas explained the need for a trained therapist. Right off, Austin's new group decided to use the $2,000 remaining in the inactive unit's coffers for the start. Then the ball began to roll: a physical occupational therapist was hired; a local church [Central Christian Church] offered its Boy Scout room (its entrance level with the sidewalk) as a temporary Center; and Austin men volunteered to make the equipment for the fledgling center. Moreover, funds from charitable enterprises were raised (at a charity ball by City Panhellenic, money from Easter Seals and financial support from the Junior League of Austin, which is now a co-sponsor of the CP Center).

During this active spring of 1948, it should be remembered that at the time when a fund-raising campaign was being staged, the new Center was holding daily sessions in that little Boy Scout room, so small that only two or three children could be cared for at one time, while others waited on the sidewalk outside. Volunteers worked on the haphazard schedule, with the mothers and other interested women sharing the duties as directed by the Center's one professional therapist.

With more financial aid coming in, the church's choir loft became the speech therapy room and the workers today can laugh about it as it was no small problem involved in carrying the crippled youngsters high into the loft for speech sessions. Dr. Jesse Villareal, top speech expert from the University of Texas, supplied much of the equipment for that first speech room.

As Bess Harris Jones took an occasional moment to reflect on her work with Austin Cerebral Palsy Center, she could not help but remember the efforts of all those who worked with her to complete the project. Certainly, she would remember the instrumental part the former Mayor, Tom Miller, played in having the new Center built. Miller persuaded the city council that "Austin indeed takes care of its own." After a search of available city property, the Council and Society officials decided upon the present site of the Cerebral Palsy Center, 919 West 28th ½ Street. The city rented the property to the Center under a rent-free, renewable 10-year lease. The building proper was provided from a $12,000 grant from the city government plus sound-proof speech room from the Lions Club, and a complete kitchen unit from Alpha Gamma Delta sorority. Howard Barr, Austin architect, voluntarily served as the architect of the new building. The Junior chamber of Commerce has added a school room to the CP Center; the Austin Kiwanis Club has added a new Physical Therapy Room. Records have been furnished free of charge to the Center; doctors serve voluntarily on the staff. The list of people who had become interested in the work of the CP Center through the efforts of Miss Jones grew each month.

All these "memories" and more are important to Bess Harris Jones's story, but the greatest tribute that can ever be paid to her is to watch the grateful eyes of the crippled youngsters and those of their parents at hope's first dawning, and on through therapy periods when hope breaks through into the joy of "marked improvement."

From the time of Harris's birth, Robin's mother, Bess, completely devoted her family and her life to this cause. She felt like she had no choice; she was on a mission to help Harris and the many other kids with CP to overcome this debilitating condition. Unfortunately, this took an unbearable toll on Bess's family, for it seemed she devoted every minute to the Austin CP Center and helping little Harris with his CP. The rest of the family took second priority. To make matters worse, in that day and age, families with kids with CP could not, or would not, share their grief openly, either because there was no support structure or because of the social norms of that day, or because talking about CP was just taboo. Many even believed that families inflicted with CP must have done something wrong or were being somehow punished by spiritual forces. Little was known back then about what caused CP; there were just a lot of theories.

Today we have learned so much more factual information about CP from pioneers such as Bess Jones and the folks at the Austin CP Center. Without Harris, it would have been highly unlikely that the Austin CP Center would have come to be. Without the Austin CP Center, many well-established protocols to treat and care for cerebral palsy would not have been discovered and made available to kids in the greater Central Texas area (and beyond), kids like me. I have a deep appreciation for Harris and his mother, Bess Jones, and I will always cherish the time I spent with Robin, reminiscing with her over stories of her mother and of the Austin CP Center.

Programs for Kids
with CP Today

BESS WAS AN EARLY PIONEER IN THE BATTLE AGAINST CP. BUT WHAT are the cutting-edge technologies today? Enter the NAPA Center, where parents can now take their children with CP. As it turns out, the NAPA Center had just opened its newest site right here in Austin a few months before my research led me to the NAPA Center. NAPA, short for Neurological and Physical Abilitation, was founded in 2008 by Lynette LaScala. Lynette spent two decades traveling around the world in search of the best therapies and treatments for her son, Cody. Cody experienced a near drowning accident on his first birthday. Cody survived; however, he developed CP.[15] Lynette made it her life's mission to help him reach his full potential and to instill hope. Her journeys around the world inspired her to make the best and most innovative therapies available under one roof for all with CP.

The NAPA Center[16] is headquartered in Los Angeles, with facilities there as well as in Sydney, Boston, Austin, and Melbourne, with more planned in the upcoming years. NAPA Center individually tailors intensive therapy programs to kids' unique needs, including cerebral palsy and other neuromuscular conditions. Their program utilizes cutting-edge technologies and new procedures that were not available during my days as a little kid at the

Austin CP Center. As I met with Lynette and the staff at the Austin NAPA Center, I became overwhelmed with joy. I was convinced that, finally, this is a fun and exciting time for kids with CP.

I continued to dig deeper into the various therapies at NAPA and was very excited to meet Lynette. What passion and drive she has for bettering the lives of kids with CP! Her son Cody has become the "Harris," while Lynette is the "Bess Jones" of today's drive to improve the lives of these most vulnerable kids.

During our many conversations, Lynette introduced me to Sarah Ross, the general manager of the Austin, Texas, center. Sarah runs the Austin site, which was opened in early 2020. She invited me to visit and meet her staff of exceptional therapists and experience what the NAPA Center is all about. Since then, I have spent many hours observing and learning all about treatments and protocols that were not available or known back in my day as a kid—such as NeuroSuits (more details later), bungee cages for teaching kids how to stand and orient to gravity, shaker tables, ESTIM treatments, and even big colorful balls for kids to balance on—all practiced at the NAPA Center. Today, speech therapists employ computer systems and technologies that can track kids' eye movements and help them learn to talk in ways that were only a dream back in the seventies. All this technology and these techniques remind me of a science fiction novel I once read as a small boy with CP. In many respects, the book has now become "science fact" in action, right in front of my eyes. I am so excited that there are programs like this for today's youngsters.

Of the many treatment plans I learned about, I was most captivated by one in particular: I witnessed kids in unique space-age-looking suits, performing tasks that reminded me of my time at the Austin CP Center. The suits were bungee-style, with supports and ties that helped them move and gain strength. They call this Napa Suit Therapy, and the little suits are called NeuroSuits.[17] This therapy is a game changer for kids with CP.

I further learned that Napa Suit Therapy, or Intensive Suit Therapy, is indeed an *intensive suit therapy treatment*[18] protocol that complements traditional therapy practices and is used to improve and increase the muscle tone, movement, posture, and motor skills of children with cerebral palsy and other neurological impairments. I found it interesting and ironic that the original therapy suit was first developed in the 1960s for cosmonauts in the Soviet space program to help prevent muscular atrophy and bone loss (osteopenia) that typically occurs when they live and work without gravity for long periods of time. Shortly after its adoption into their space program, Soviet researchers introduced and tested a modified version of this original "space-age" suit as a physical therapy device for children with neurological disorders like CP.

These form-fitting, segmented suits are attached with straps and strong elastic cords that support the body and create resistance to movements. Adjustments can be made to generate various tensions on major muscle groups. The tension places pressure on joints to correct muscle alignment, improve proprioception (the ability to sense the position, location, orientation, and movement of the body and its various parts), strengthen muscles, enhance sensory awareness, and treat a wide range of neurological disorders that manifest as a lack of motor control. The NAPA Center has integrated the NeuroSuit and Intensive Suit Therapy into its program.[19]

Intensive Suit Therapy accomplishes three things: it loads, compresses, and aligns.[20]

1. Loads—the suit can load up to forty pounds of directed pressure to the body to activate the antigravity muscles of the body, namely, the muscles that get you up off the ground to crawl, stand, jump, walk, and run.

2. Compresses—a compression suit acts as a girdle of support for body awareness. It is important to promote proper body awareness to our systems. If you don't know where your body is in relationship to other objects, to other people, or to the greater world, you will never be able to move through the world efficiently.

3. Aligns—the therapy activates alignment muscles to help engage the underlying musculature and promote better posture and body alignment. If your body is not in the right place to begin with, it doesn't matter if you can turn on the muscles or not, because the muscles will not be able to do the right thing.

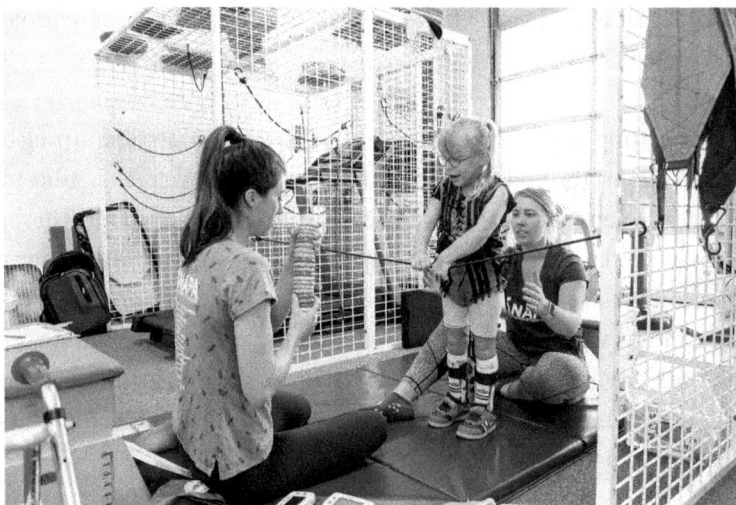

Intensive Suit Therapy treatment protocol in the bungee cage

Due to the history of this suit with cosmonauts, I imagine there is also a version of the NeuroSuit for adults with CP, but since most current research and programs end at the age of thirteen, I have not been able to find one.

Moreover, as part of my research, my personal transformation, and writing this book, I have come to follow several kids with CP who have had significant success through the NAPA program. The program includes the NeuroSuit and boasts powerful stories that just melt my heart. I like to imagine that's where the big colorful ball I used in my treatment plan ended up, helping kids like me succeed in life, thanks to the NAPA Center (but I'm getting ahead of myself here).

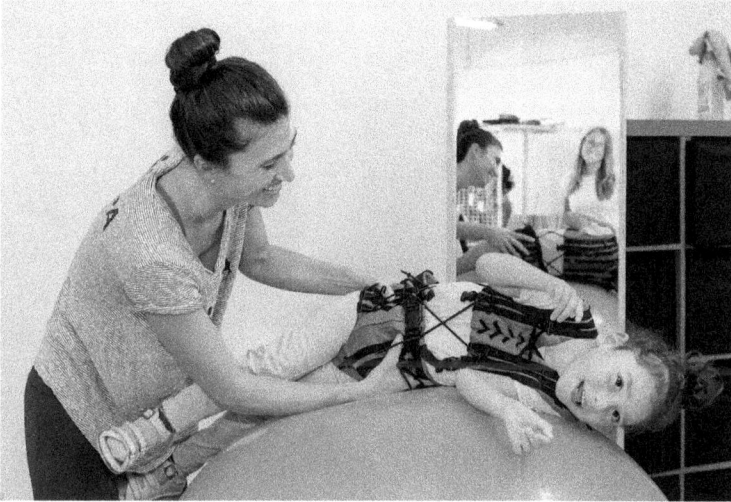

Both Bess and Lynette have a passion for helping those with CP. I share this same trait, with an added benefit: I have firsthand experience of not only having CP but overcoming CP's various limitations. Like Bess and Lynette, I too want to help those with CP by sharing my successes. I want to help provide inspiration, motivation, and most importantly, hope to those just starting out on their own transformations.

With that said, let's start at the beginning of my story. The story of something "spectacularly amazing" (a refrain I'd use often during my difficult physical training).

PART 2

Beginnings

His Timing Is Always Perfect

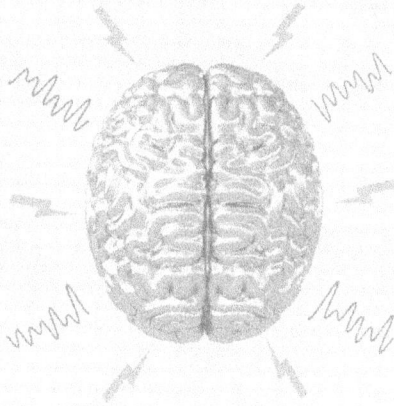

Adopted in Love

I was born July 3, 1967, at 9:25 p.m. in Fort Worth, Texas, four weeks premature. I had a rough start, weighing in at only five pounds, five ounces, and eighteen inches long—early to my own birth but late to almost every life experience thereafter. I guess that's why today I am somewhat paranoid about being late for anything. Deep down in my subconscious, I must be anxious about missing out on something amazing.

I started out in this world stripped from my birth mother and placed for adoption by the Volunteers of America adoption program, a nonprofit ministry that transforms lives by reaching and uplifting America's most vulnerable. I never found out much about my maternal or paternal history. My adopted mom and dad wrote down a few things in a somewhat frantic fashion during one of many visits with the agency, and I later made multiple requests for information from the Texas Department of Health, which provided heavily redacted responses.

However, I was never able to find any medical or family genetic history. Today, genetics seems to be the hot topic of conversation around family dinner tables, but back in the early seventies, this was certainly not the case. My genetic history was simply unknown, and as I grew up, I was told *there was no way I could find out where I came from*. But still I often wondered what my birth family was like.

My parents started the adoption process three years before I was born. I guess the process for matching, adoption, and actual placement can be long and drawn out, or at least it was back then. It turned out that I was a perfect fit for their new family.

I was told that my birth was normal for the most part. However, it was recorded that I had experienced a forceps rotation delivery that affected my atlas vertebra. The atlas, also known as C1, is the topmost vertebra of the spinal column. It is in direct contact with the occipital bone, a flat bone located at the back portion of the head. This means that the medical staff used forceps or, as I was told as a small kid, "salad tongs," to pull me out by my head, turning my head to get me "unstuck." *Really?* The thought still makes me cringe to this day.

Since I was a preemie, I had to wait in the neonatal intensive care unit (NICU) to make sure I was gaining enough weight before I could go to my new home. Everything about those early years in Austin seemed to go well, until I was about eighteen months old. At that point, my parents noticed I did not reach for toys with my right hand. That's when my pediatrician, Dr. Willburn, gave me a label that would forever change the course of my life and cause more trouble than it seemed to solve. He told my mom and dad that I was developing slowly on my right side because of a type of brain damage known as spastic hemiplegic cerebral palsy.[21]

As mentioned above, hemiplegic CP, or unilateral CP, affects the movement and muscle tone on one side of the body. This is the most common form of CP, with estimates ranging from 33 to 40 percent of all people with cerebral palsy. Most often this is caused by a neonatal stroke in the time before, during, or slightly after birth due to lack of oxygen to the brain. Multiple factors may interact to block the blood vessels in or to the brain, which causes a stroke. Many times, as in my case, the exact cause of the stroke will never be known. However, the forceps and turning of my head most likely contributed to the cause. As one side of the brain is injured, the opposite side of the body is affected; this can result in weakness of an arm, leg, or both on one side of the body. It is said that 60 percent of children with hemiplegic CP have seizures during this newborn period.

In my case, CP affected my entire right side, including my hand, arm, leg, and foot. It was a while after I was born before we learned that it also affected the speech and balance centers of my brain. The good news was that I did not experience seizures. Specifically, my little baby right arm would not extend, and my right hand was all fisted-up in an abducted state and would not reach and grab objects like my left hand would. My right foot and leg were also not properly aligned, and my right hip joint tendons and ligaments were not yet strong enough to maintain proper alignment, causing my right foot to pronate and point outward. In layman's terms, my knee was turning out, causing my heel to turn in and toes to point out. Later on, I developed a condition I came to dread, called "spasticity," where certain affected muscles are continuously involuntarily contracted. In my case, this contraction caused stiffness or tightness of the muscles and interfered with normal movement. This is most notably seen in walking; my gait became an abnormal toe-heel, toe-heel pattern on my right side and a normal, relaxed heel-toe, heel-toe pattern on my left. Furthermore, my right arm curled up near my chest, and my right hand balled up in a bent fist.

As a child, I went through many tests that must have made me look like Frankenstein's baby. I had wires and electrical gizmos everywhere. Two tests in particular stuck out to me—positron emission tomography (PET) scans and computerized tomography (CAT or CT) scans. As a tot, I loved animals, but I never saw any cats or pets in the doctor's office or hospitals I was in—just wires all over my head and tiny body. You name it—if a test was available in 1968, I likely experienced it. The end results showed I had around 2 to 3 percent brain damage in the left hemisphere, confirming their diagnosis of spastic hemiplegic cerebral palsy. Although the GMFCS rating system was not developed until 1997, I have extrapolated that I would have been classified as GMFCS Level II. I am using the classification here as a retrospective measurement.[22] Needless to say, CP was a label that I would soon learn to hate growing up.

Against my dad's advice, Mom took me to an osteopath in Fort Worth. Dr. Ellis performed one chiropractic treatment, free of charge because I was just a baby, to correct a subluxation of my cervical spine at C3 and C4, correcting what my other doctors referred to as "a nervous system disturbance, which was causing the neurological interference." This one little adjustment opened up blood flow to my right arm. Mom told me that at the exact moment of treatment, she saw color "return" to my right arm and hand while blood moved into the veins of my right arm, and immediately after his adjustment, my right fist opened up for the first time. She could not wait to have my dad trim my right fingernails later on that evening. For my parents, trimming my fingernails was a task that was futile at worst and exceedingly difficult at best. She was anxious for my father to see me extend my right arm and open my right hand. He was indeed amazed but still a bit skeptical and did not like the idea that I had gone to a chiropractor.

THE EARLY YEARS

When I was just a little tot, from age two to six years old, Mom took me across town five days a week to the Austin CP Center off of West 28th ½ Street, where I learned life skills while the therapists worked on my body.

I was timid at first and did not want to be separated from Mom. Every day I would get to explore and play around in a room that had lots of interesting toys, a big ball to roll around on, and parallel bars to help kids like me walk. On one side, there was a huge mirror that ran the entire length of the room. I guessed it was there so we could see ourselves playing. I got to spend time with several genuinely nice therapists.

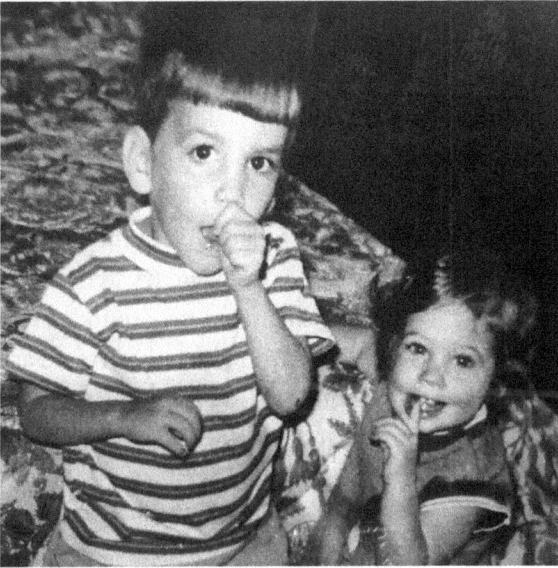

With my younger sister, Karen

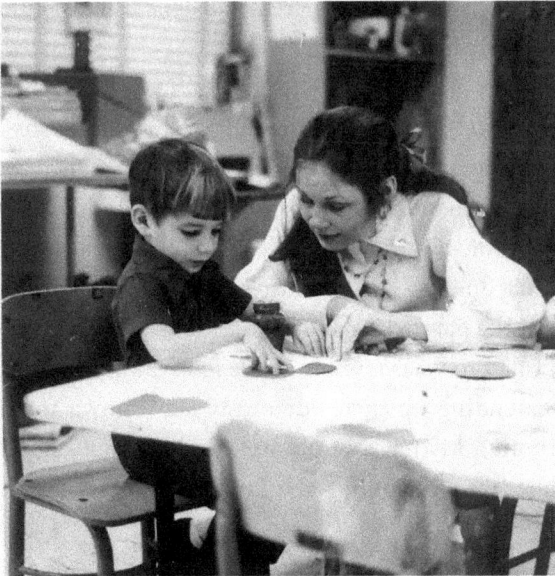

*Learning right-hand tactile skills at the
Austin CP Center, circa 1972*

One in particular, Jamie Tucker, would work with me a lot. I remember liking her. One of my favorite things was when my therapist would hold my feet and roll me around on top of a giant, inflated stability ball that had different-colored stripes on it. She would ask me to lie on top of the red stripe, and I would find the red stripe and lay my skinny belly down and wait for her to grab my feet. While she held my feet and rolled me around on this ball, I would extend my arms over my head as best I could and try to reach the floor, which seemed far, far below my head. As she rolled me around, I would imagine I was floating in space. She would tell me to touch the ground as she rolled me toward the floor, but I was never quite able to reach the ground with my right hand. I would lie on my stomach and on my back, rolling from side to side or forward and backward. Sometimes I would even get to sit up, and she would hold my feet and arms as she rolled me around on top of this big ball. But my best memories were rolling around on my belly with my arms stretched out like Mighty Mouse. Only years later did I learn that all this ball work was designed to help me with my inner-ear balance receptors and the spatial aptitude centers of my brain. Learning where my body was in relationship to the earth would ultimately lead to increased balance and walking ability. They called this fun stuff "physical therapy."

I would also learn to walk better using the parallel bars at the far end of the room. Using my hands to hold the brown wooden rails, I would practice walking heel-toe, heel-toe, with my shoes on at first, then later barefoot. In the beginning, it was hard for me to grip the bar with my right hand and hold myself stable due to a lack of muscle tone on my right side, but as I got older, walking at the parallel bars seemed to get easier. When I wasn't in this special room, I had to wear an ugly black shoe on my right foot with thick metal braces extending up each side of my leg (known today as an AFO: ankle foot orthotic). My left foot did not need a brace, only the ugly black shoe. These shoes were uncomfortable, and my right foot always hurt when I wore them.

I also remember wearing a metal brace between my legs at night. The brace had a bar near my ankles, attached to both legs, preventing my right leg from rotating out or in or bending my knee. I could not move or walk in this metal confinement. All I could do was lie there and wonder why I had to endure all this. It was like I had a cast on both legs, and I could only lie flat on my back. Years later I would learn that this bar and brace were used to help my right hip socket develop properly, as the muscles and tendons were too weak and stiff to hold my right leg and foot in proper alignment while sleeping in a relaxed position.

Some of my occupational therapy consisted of learning to dress and undress with both hands, which included buttoning my shirt. This may sound simple enough, but for a kid with CP, it was a huge ordeal. Before my therapy began, I was not using my right hand and arm at all, not even as a "helper" hand. It was hard to dress and undress as a youngster, using only one functioning hand and arm.

At the CP Center, I started out working with strips of fabric with large buttons, then graduated to buttoning my own shirt. Mom would bring all sorts of clothes from home. My pajamas were an item of particular interest to my therapists, as I recall. I would repeatedly dress and undress. Put on my pjs and then take off my pjs. Then put my play clothes back on, including my socks and shoes. This was not only frustrating as a tactile and dexterity exercise, but also, I didn't understand *why* I had to keep dressing and undressing all the time. *Why couldn't the grown-ups make up their minds as to what I should wear?* Since my right arm wouldn't extend all the way and my right hand wouldn't grip, my shirt was the hardest to take off, and I found all this activity quite frustrating as a kid.

During the winter months, my therapists taught me a special way to put on my coat. I would spread out my coat on a bed with the zipper unzipped, facing down, collar facing away from me, with the arms extended to each side. Then I would walk up to my coat, stick both arms in the arm holes, and work my hands all the way to the ends of each hole. I would then lift my arms as high as I could and tuck my chin down as low as I could. Usually, the coat would slide down over my head and down my backside, and like magic, my coat was on.

But on some occasions, my coat would get stuck over my head or somewhere on my backside, and I would have to wiggle out of my self-imposed straitjacket and start all over again.

I learned how to tie my shoes with my laces in a bow, just like Mom would do for me. It always impressed me when she would tie them so fast. For me, it felt like trying to tie wet angel-hair pasta with butter on my hands. It was frustrating. But with practice, I learned to wrap my right shoelace around my right thumb, then grip it in my right hand, moving the shoelace around with my left hand while my right was stationary, still gripping the lace as tight as I could. Over, under, around, through, then pull tight. That was the *first* part of my knot. Then came the harder part: the bow. Again, grip the end with my right, as before. Around, through, and then pull evenly with both hands. Usually, I would have to do it all over again because the first knot had wiggled loose while I was working on the pasta bow, or I would lose the grip with my right hand.

At the CP Center, I also learned activities such as placing squares into square holes, round pegs into round holes, and stars into star-shaped holes, using my right hand. My left hand even got a turn at this game. My left hand usually won these internal competitions; I always wanted to use my left hand, and my therapist would quickly remind me to use my right. To me, it was a hassle and a complete waste of time. The fingers on my right hand wouldn't do what I wanted them to do. Moreover, I wanted to get the game over with so I could return to my big colorful ball and be Mighty Mouse once more.

Early on during my research of the Austin CP Center, my mother shared with me a note she wrote many years back. This note was her account of what it was like to take me to the Austin CP Center and what activities I did. She told me she attended every one of my sessions, observing everything. Here is her written account of my sessions:

> We went to the Austin CP Center five mornings a week and Scott would
> have 30 minutes of physical therapy, 30 minutes of speech and 30 more

minutes of occupational therapy. Physical therapy was straightforward: Scott was on a table and the therapist would manipulate his limbs. In contrast, Speech therapy dealt with developmentally appropriate sounds, blends and putting them together to make words.

There was a range of activities in the occupational block—everything from lightly brushing Scott's right arm with a soft brush, which always seemed to intrigue him…to getting him to use his right hand during several weeks of dressing classes. The brushing movements were to stimulate his sense and touch receptors and reinforce positive neuro-feedback. Dressing class was the most frustrating; it required dexterity and small movements to button and unbutton, work zippers, tie and untie shoelaces, put shoes on the right feet, and put on and take off clothes, PJs, and a coat or jacket. Scott never quite mastered the zipper, so the Center introduced Scott to a new product called Velcro.

During these days, many tears were shed in this process—both Scott's and mine.

RIP GOES THE WEASEL:
STORIES OF GROWING UP WITH CP

Back when I was a little tot at the Austin CP Center, Mom wanted to dress me in pull-up type pants, but I really wanted my own pair of blue jeans, just like the other kids had. At the CP Center, they tried to teach me how to zip up my brand-new jeans, but my right hand and fingers were just too weak, and I did not have the dexterity to hold that tiny metal zipper handle.

The sound of Velcro is easy to recognize today, but back in the early seventies, Velcro was not common at all.

Velcro was the creation of Swiss engineer and inventor George de Mestral,[23] who discovered this "burr" product by happenstance during a hike in the

Jura Mountains with his dog in 1941. De Mestral noticed that burrs from the burdock plant had attached themselves to his pants and to his trusty dog's fur. How could so small an object exert such a stronghold? Under the microscope, de Mestral could see that the tips of the burr contained tiny hooks that could attach themselves to fibers in clothing, similar to a hook-and-eye fastener.

De Mestral knew that if he could somehow recreate the burr's simple hook system, he would be able to produce an incredibly strong fastener.

He spent the next fourteen years attempting to duplicate what he saw under that microscope before finally introducing it to the world in 1955. De Mestral called his new product "Velcro," from the French words *velour* (velvet) and *crochet* (hook).

As an interesting sidenote, Velcro was used during the Apollo missions to anchor equipment for astronauts' convenience in zero-gravity situations. So why not use this material for my zipper problem?

I bet de Mestral never thought his Velcro would help kids with CP.

My therapists' bright idea, to sew black Velcro over my pants zipper, was intended to allow me to grab my zipper flap and pull apart my pants with confidence and ease. However, the loud noise it made became another issue altogether. Every pair of my jeans and shorts that had a zipper was quickly reinforced with this very loud space-age product called Velcro.

Over time, however, I became very conscious of what Velcro sounded like in the restroom. While in my stall or standing at attention…suddenly everybody would hear a loud "RIPPPP" from the next stall. It was embarrassing to walk out of my stall or away from a urinal afterward, toward all those people who must have wondered what the sound was and if I was feeling all right. As a kid with CP, the Velcro drew even more unwanted attention my way. I still remember hearing the murmurs: "What's wrong with that boy?"

I did try to "rip" my pants slowly and quietly, but when nature calls, this slow pace would not always work, and I would have to rip my fly open in a hurry—only to hear that loud ripping sound again, echoing off the interior walls of the bathroom.

I had Velcro sewn into my pants until I was in the fifth grade. My first pair of jeans with a button fly was total heaven to me, even if Mom had to widen the buttonholes slightly to make them easier for me to operate. For the first time, I was able to go to the restroom in pure silence. Using zippers came much later as I adapted and learned to reverse my left and right hands to operate. My stronger left hand would grasp the tiny zipper handle while my right would act as an anchor to either pull or push against the zipper. Today, the modified "zipper role reversal" technique is so ingrained in my muscle memory that I have to fight not to employ it, even though I am now able to operate zippers properly. Needless to say, every time I hear the sound of Velcro, my attention is momentarily drawn to past memories of my distant youth.

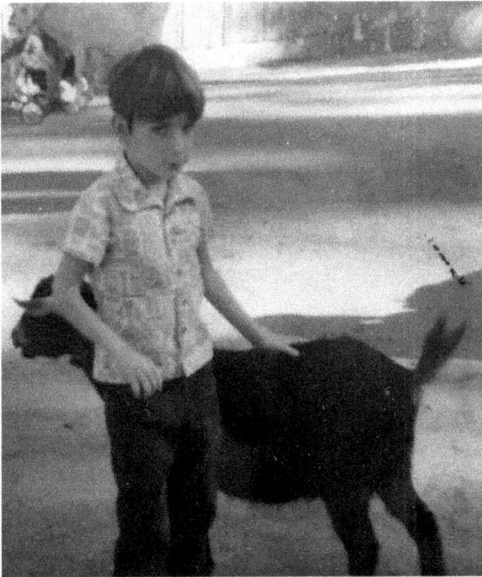

Scared and timid at the Austin Zoo

At the CP Center, I got to hang out with three other kids my age who also had CP: Gavin, Paul, and Cindy. We became fast friends and hung out together a lot. Our parents formed a support group and would get together while we were in our sessions at the CP Center or would hang out at our lake house, where I lived as a kid. Our parents ended up creating our own little support group both for us kids and for our parents to deal with the constant strain of having a child with CP. We three would play in the water, ride around in Dad's ski boat, and just be kids. Since we all had CP, we felt normal together.

Toward the end of my time at the CP Center, I remember holding my mom's hand as we entered a dark room next to my playroom. I don't remember why I was with her and not on my favorite ball next door. She talked to the doctors and the therapist as we entered. All the lights were off in this room, and a few grown-ups were looking out of a big, long window. After the door closed behind me and my eyes adjusted to the darkness, I saw what everyone was looking at: it was my playroom with my big, round colorful ball! Why were these people looking out the window into my playroom, and why were there windows in my room when it was a mirror on the other side? No one explained any of this to me, and I was very confused. After that day, I never saw that big glass mirror quite the same again. In fact, to this day, I look at mirrors with a raised eyebrow. *Who is looking in on me and why?* Decades later, I would learn that this room was an observation room for parents and doctors to watch kids during occupational and physical therapy sessions. Mom told me that she would watch every session, and the doctors would track my progress from there.

Shortly after my seventh birthday, in 1973, we moved to the Eanes Independent School District, where I began first grade, and I stopped going to the Austin CP Center. I always assumed that the CP Center had closed its doors.

When I followed up with Robin Cooper, I discovered that when Harris was older, Bess gave birth to a healthy baby boy named Mark. Bess was unable to simultaneously take care of both boys, so Harris Jones was moved and admitted to the Austin State School for round-the-clock care, something that the

Austin CP Center could not provide. As a result, Bess shifted her focus from the Austin CP Center to programs at the Austin State School. Soon after, in 1974, the Austin CP Center became the Capital Area Rehabilitation Center (CARC). In 1985, the CP Center became an official affiliate of the Easter Seals and was renamed the Capital Area Easter Seals Society. Then, in 1998, the name was changed to Easter Seals Central Texas (ESCT). In 2010, there were more changes as ESCT expanded to include more comprehensive community and housing services.

The organization has since changed its name to Easterseals Central Texas and now provides services to more than 8,500 patients and families from the region. However, as a small kid growing into adolescence, I wondered why such a wonderful place for kids with CP would be shut down. *What about the kids like me who needed help like I received?* I wondered for years. As it turns out, I had just moved on to a new environment, like Harris had.

As I started grade school west of Austin, I began to see a new therapist. However, I do not remember excelling like I did at the Austin CP Center. In fact, I did not excel as I did during those earlier years at all. I just wondered about the other kids like me. And more importantly, what ever happened to my big, round colorful ball? I bet it ended up at the NAPA Center.

Leo Goes to School

Leo the Late Bloomer by Robert Kraus was my favorite book, or rather the only book I wanted Mom to read to me as a toddler.[24] This thirty-two-page book is about a little lion named Leo who is not reading, writing, drawing, or even speaking, and everyone is concerned. Everyone except his mom, that is. She knows her son is a lion and that he will do all those things and more when he's ready. Leo seems to be late at everything. It's sort of poetic that this became my favorite. Mom said that every time we would go to the Austin Public Library, I would pick only that book. She had practically memorized it, reading to me every night before bedtime. *Would Leo be my role model in life to come? Was I Leo the Lion with CP?*

Growing up in Eanes, an affluent upper-middle-class school district west of Austin in West Lake Hills, I found school to be quite difficult. This district has been home to some extraordinarily talented athletes over many years. It's highly rated in sports as well as academia. In fact, I would say that it's intensely focused on sports perfection, and this was extremely hard to overcome for a boy like me. By first grade, I was a skinny, wiry, and very, very shy youngster—not exactly a model for any sports megastar or even a contender in physical education class. As a coping mechanism, I fast became an introverted kid—partly as a result of my cerebral palsy and partly due to a lack of understanding. I didn't get why other kids could be so cruel to kids like me, kids who were "less than normal."

A lot of kids with CP develop an extremely low self-esteem early on due to a societal lack of understanding (from kids in particular). Coupled with me "becoming" the Leo of Robert Kraus's book, my self-esteem was in trouble. I became paralyzed with a fear of failure, and I began to withdraw from learning about healthy competition and socialization skills (team sports) as a kid.

In sports like dodgeball, I was usually the last one to be picked for a team and one of the first to feel the business end of that fast-moving, unpredictable red ball. In games like softball, I actually prayed for our team to strike out before my turn because I did not know how to swing a bat and connect with that tiny white ball traveling toward me with such velocity, taunting me as it passed by my head. Kickball was a little better. My left foot could connect with the ball with an accuracy I didn't know I possessed. I would kick the ball with my left foot without losing balance on my right, then begin running for what seemed like a mile to first base. From there, it was just a matter of keeping focus on who was at home plate kicking the next ball…and on when the kid on second began his run so I could then run to second base. Oftentimes I would get the timing all wrong and get boxed in between first base and the runner who was still on second base. Oh my! This game was so confusing, and I could hear the kids laughing at me.

Every year in PE, we all had to perform something called the Presidential Fitness Test, followed by Sports Day, an Olympic-style sports competition. The Presidential Fitness Test included push-ups, pull-ups, sit-ups, and timed running skill tests. For me and my weak right side, push-ups were all but impossible. This did not stop my PE coaches from humiliating me in front of the entire class. I would have to get on all fours and attempt a full bridged push-up. They didn't seem to understand the concept of my CP. Heck, I didn't understand it, and I had it. All they said was, "Scott, get your nose off the dirt and give me ten."

Oh, right Coach, I thought. *After I figure out how to do my first one, I'll get right on those other nine.*

I spent a lot of time with my nose buried in that dry, dusty dirt on the upper sports field at Eanes Elementary, trying my best to do an unbalanced push-up with my left side, unable to fully compensate for my weaker right side, with very little core strength at all. To this day, when I assume that push-up position, I experience Sports Day PTSD. Little did those coaches know, their treatment was so counterproductive that it drove me to quit. For a long time, I stopped trying at *any* sport at *any* cost.

Back in those days, you did not hear words like *core* or *trunk* or even *abdominals*. We just knew we had to have a tight stomach, strong back, and strong arms to do things right. With my cerebral palsy, my stomach and back muscles were *not* strong, and my coaches did nothing to try and fix this deficiency. Sit-ups were okay, as long as someone was sitting on my feet to keep them on the ground. Back then, we had to come all the way up and touch elbows to knees, so I got to rest for a microsecond on each rep. To rest even more, I used the excuse of trying to get my right elbow to my right knee. This was a hassle in itself, however. I could only do a dozen or so before tiring out. Pull-ups were like push-ups since they required both arms to perform properly. I remember that just trying to hold on with my right hand was hard enough. Staring at the bar and trying to pull myself up to what seemed like an infinite distance was like trying to do the Jedi mind trick on your teacher to get out of work. Trust me when I say that it does not work. We did not know about wrist straps or hand grips back then, so I could barely hang on, much less pull up my body weight—and when I tried, I would swing to my stronger left side. My right hand was unable to maintain its grip; it would let go of the bar altogether and curl up to my chest while my left hand hung on for dear life. All the kids would laugh, and they called me names like "monkey-boy" and other names that were cruel for anyone, much less a shy kid with CP.

My cerebral palsy affected my right foot and leg as well. Even though I no longer used my special shoe with rods (AFOs), CP caused me to walk funny, and as a result, I favored my stronger left side. I would walk with a spastic toe-heel, toe-heel step on my right and a proper, relaxed heel-toe, heel-toe step on my left, with a pronounced gimpy-limp. By then, my left calf was starting to overcompensate and become larger than my right calf. I imagined that this made my legs look like half penguin, half elephant when I walked or wobbled.

The simple dynamics of walking were hard. But running was a whole different dynamic. I was surprisingly good at running and sprinting due to my toe-heel, toe-heel walk on my right side. After all, sprinters run on their toes. This was cool. I could actually run on my toes very well.

Dr. Karen Pape writes about running and walking with CP in her book, *The Boy Who Could Run but Not Walk.*[25] She explains that running is a higher-learned skill, usually developed later, after a CP-inflicted kid's brain damage had healed. In my case, my neuromuscular pathways for running developed later in childhood, after my brain had had the time it needed to heal, so there was not an "inefficient" (maladaptive) neuromuscular pathway established earlier, like that for walking. The spasticity that I endured while walking seemed to lessen while I ran. Endurance was yet another issue.

Due to a lack of physical fitness and stamina, I would tire easily. I did better with sprinting shorter distances. Unfortunately, the distances I usually ran were a bit farther than I was comfortable with at any sprint speed. I still cringe whenever I hear the term *five-hundred-meter dash* or *eight-hundred-meter sprint.* Apparently, there were no sprinting distances with obtainable good run times for a kid like me. These distances all took stamina and pacing, concepts no one had taught me as a kid. So the timed runs were nothing more than failure waiting for me at the finish line.

I found that it was easier and less humiliating to just forgo participating in sports. Unfortunately, this became the norm for me on the playground and beyond. I learned, "Do not try, and you will not fail," better known today as the "flight response." This became my sports motto. Leo was not learning sports for a long time. Leo was in for a ride.

This learned response followed me academically as well, resulting in me quickly falling behind in the classroom. A "Do not attempt, and I will not fail" mentality was firmly ingrained in almost everything I did. I did not under-stand how important learning was back then. I don't know if cerebral palsy caused a learning disability or if using empathy and sympathy along with this avoidance tactic caused me to lag behind in my coursework, thus resulting in my slow learning. This theory needs more research as a whole. However, as I study empathy and avoidance with regards to CP, my educated and personal assessment makes me lean toward CP not causing my learning disability but rather contributing to my learning at a slower pace. I believe this was a direct result of me picking up on the adults around me having a bias toward kids with CP not being as smart as normal kids. This is inaccurate, but it existed nonetheless. Basically, it is the classic causality principle in action. Because people treated me like I had a learning disability, I believed I had a learning disability, and consequently, it became true. A self-fulfilling prophecy.

By my third-grade year, my ploys for getting out of schoolwork with the aid of empathy and sympathy ended abruptly when I was introduced to a very astute special education resource teacher by the name of Mrs. Sandy Jenkins. This one teacher would forever change the trajectory of my life and ultimately spark my love for learning in the years to come. She put an end to the tactics I had been employing to get out of doing schoolwork.

By this point in my early academic career, my sister, Karen, and I were attend-ing an after-school program called Lamplighter every day until 5:00 p.m. Mom would then pick us up after she got off work. Lamplighter was right down the street from Eanes Elementary, so my sister and I would walk there with an escort after school at 3:30 p.m. and play until Mom came. Sandy called the house one evening and said she wanted to start keeping me after school to drill me on "math facts." She would take me home once I had mastered what she had planned for each evening. This would continue after each school day until I was up to her standards. That first day with her, I did not leave for home till 7:30 p.m.

Mom said when I arrived home that first day, I was exhausted and starving. I ate a late supper and went straight to bed with no motherly prompting. The second day, I stayed until 6:00 p.m. By the third day, I made it home around 5:00 p.m. For those three days, I stayed after school with Sandy, listening to soft classical music, doing my assigned homework, and practicing my math. Then I returned home by way of the "Sandy sports-car ride," always hungry and tired.

On one occasion, Mrs. Jenkins told Mom that I liked classical music and perhaps my mom could play it for me at home, as study music. Today, every time I hear Beethoven or Bach, I have disturbing flashbacks of those after-school sessions in Mrs. Jenkins's study chamber. It was indeed a psychological battle of spirit and will, and she was committed to breaking me like a wild horse—at all costs. By day three, however, Mrs. Jenkins allowed me to return to Lamplighter after school with no more follow-on after-school sessions. To this day, I still wonder who won.

By the fifth grade, I was at a new school, Cedar Creek Elementary. Ironically, Mrs. Jenkins had decided to transfer to my new school as well, to follow my progress and remain at the helm, steering my USS *Learning*. Cedar Creek was a brand-new school in the Eanes district for third through fifth graders. We were even issued "Eagle Cards" that we used to get into school events and as hall passes. I finagled two cards so that when one was confiscated due to "mischief," I still had my "get out of jail free" card.

My special education math class met up in a loft area above the library called the Eagle's Nest and was taught by none other than Mrs. Jenkins. Apparently, I was still dead center on her sonar. At the beginning of each class, for about twenty minutes, she would put me in a dark closet on the left side of the nest with another student. The other student would "drill me" on my multiplication tables, loud enough for Mrs. Jenkins and the rest of the class to hear on the other side of the door. She instructed the other student to leave the light off so I'd have no opportunity to use any form of cheating material. I could only imagine the fear this instilled in my "drillmaster" in the closet with me, as well as the other members of that class who had to endure my confinement sessions every week. It was humiliating to us both and led to endless teasing after class by the other students. To this day, I vividly remember every one of those closet sessions and who was assigned to drill me each time. It's hard to admit that I did actually learn a thing or two from both the after-school detention and these various closet isolation "study" sessions.

Mrs. Jenkins rode me hard from the third grade up to the sixth grade, where she handed the teaching baton to another resource teacher, Ms. Diana Sledge, who continued this practice up through the eighth grade at Hill Country Middle School. Mrs. Jenkins was determined to break me of "my evil habits" and teach me how to learn without failure. This was a tough task for any teacher dealing with a kid with cerebral palsy who had a serious lack of motivation to learn. After all, at this point of my young life, I didn't have the belief or knowledge that I could succeed at anything.

I must admit, I did not like Mrs. Jenkins during those years, but today I am grateful she taught me unique techniques to not only help me stay afloat academically, but also to succeed in academic life by becoming an avid life-long learner, understanding and employing various methods to learn. Success and achievement are the result of novel ways of performing hard work.

FITTING IN

Everybody wants to fit in at school, even shy and introverted kids with CP like me. Up to this point in my very young academic career, I was almost completely shut off from "normal kids" in "normal" classrooms. I was locked away with other "special" kids in a classroom called "Resource."

In seventh grade, I was somewhat paroled, at least for one class. I felt I had hit the big time. I finally got to experience classes that I had only heard about from my "normal" friends on the playground.

I grew to love writing, reading, and everything that the other kids learned to do. I secretly longed to attend all those classes that the "normal kids" got to be in. I loved every minute of it…well, except maybe spelling quizzes. I would receive a list of ten words each week and sit at the table with Mom, memorizing the words by writing down the correct spelling of each one, over and over again. It was very frustrating, however, because I could not quite master how to spell. I've been told I'm a phonetic speller; apparently English is not a phonetic language. I remember trying to explain to my language arts teacher that one day there would be a way for kids to use a device to help spell words for them. I guess she was not buying what I was selling because one day after class, I overheard my mom, my resource teacher advocate (Ms. Diana Sledge), and my language arts teacher in the hallway discussing sending me back to the "special" room. Ms. Language Arts wanted me to leave her class and go back to Resource because I was unable to meet her standards in spelling.

"Scott performs everything else at grade level," my mother had said.

My resource teacher then replied that perhaps my spelling quizzes would not count and that I could work on spelling with her after class.

Ms. L. A. countered, "It would not be fair to the other students if Scott stayed in my class and received special treatment." After all, these were the days before any sort of Americans with Disabilities Act legislation.

The conversation seemed to last for an awfully long time. Or at least a long time for any seventh grader to stand. I lowered my head in defeat and returned to the very last real classroom seat I would have, and I sat and waited for my parole to end. It was going to be back to the special room for me.

However, that day never came. Thanks to my mom and my resource teacher, who both fought extremely hard on my behalf, we won the fight to keep me in regular class. Language arts actually ended up being my favorite class in seventh grade. Oh yeah, and I was correct. Ms. Language Arts should have bought what I said about "spellers." We now have spellers to help kids with spelling, which are standard on almost every electronic texting device today (even if we don't employ them correctly). I vividly remember receiving a Franklin speller soon after to help me spell. I still have that one-line LCD display Franklin as a trusty friend and a trophy for triumph in seventh-grade language arts class. I ended up joining other regular classes after that and started to feel more like I could hang with smart, normal kids.

In eighth grade I found a new interest: programming computers. I took a computer science class with Mr. Mokrey and actually earned an A. After school every day, I would stay till 5:30 p.m., programming Commodore PET and Apple II computers. I was usually the last one out of the building, so the teacher ended up giving me a key to lock up the lab when I was finished. Wow, an eighth grader with CP with a key to the school! How cool was that?

Yet when I moved on to high school, academics seemed to turn back toward failure. I was in a couple of normal classes, but the rest were back in the resource room for the most part. Unfortunately, I did not have an advocate during the high school years. Once again, I fell behind and got lost in "the system," and there were no computers to program. I also remember receiving the message loud and clear that I was not smart enough to go to college. This must be what they mean today when they talk about marginalizing kids who don't know how to perform to academic standards. Lack of hope for academic success led to the lack of motivation to even try.

I was once again in full-time flight mode. This further reinforced my younger memories of the "Do not try, and you will not fail" mindset. Why *were* there no advocates for kids like me in high school? Where were the Sandy Jenkinses now?

While my friends were off preparing to take SATs and college entrance aptitude exams, I was stuck in limbo, stuck in the resource room. *What was Leo to do after graduation?*

WATER, WATER EVERYWHERE

In addition to academics, sports continued to present challenges for me throughout my childhood. I had learned early in life to get out of every PE-related activity that I could so I wouldn't have to be embarrassed or teased by other kids. Besides, sports were so confusing to me. Team sports were the worst. I don't remember ever being introduced to traditional sports at home either. I don't know if it was because my father didn't think that I could handle sports, or because I really didn't understand the rules, or perhaps because of the lack of coordination caused by cerebral palsy. Or maybe an "I can't, so why try?" mentality so ingrained in me as a child.

All I really knew was water: being in the water or being in a competition ski boat at water-ski tournaments. I grew up in a competitive water-skiing family on Lake Austin, and I learned how to swim before I could even walk. Mom would take me down to the local swim center for swim lessons when I was just a toddler. I think that because I was always around the water, my folks wanted to make sure that I'd be able to handle myself if ever I were suddenly immersed in this alien liquid at such an early age. I would often joke that I had to learn how to swim because my parents didn't want to lose me after all that trouble of adopting me. Besides, leaving a boat by way of "man overboard" at high speed is scary enough. And yes, when I was an older kid, this was something that my *Naval Commander* dad insisted we master like a military drill at sea. Surprisingly, I fell right into it very well.

I ended up taking to water like a fish. Water, it seems, equalizes gravitational forces upon the body. This wonderful liquid permitted me to thrive and grow with cerebral palsy. I would later learn that aquatic activities improve muscle tone, strength, and muscle coordination for kids and adults with cerebral palsy.

In the book I mentioned earlier, *The Boy Who Could Run but Not Walk*, Dr. Karen Pape wrote about the remarkable therapeutic possibilities of water, and she developed a water exercise program using the Wet Vest, a neutral buoyancy device that allows children and adults to walk and jog in deep water with their heads safely out of the water. A competitive runner first developed this technique to help him recover after a war injury. The Wet Vest is now widely used in the rehabilitation of professional athletes and US military personnel.

Dr. Pape wrote, "For the child or adult with neurological problems, this is an inexpensive, effective way of providing access to out-of-gravity exercise. Learning how to stay upright and then move about a pool is a novel challenge that rapidly took the child 'out of habit' and revealed underlying recovery."[26] Dr. Pape found that it was not unusual to have "a child who walks with difficulty learn to jog in the water within minutes, moving on all four limbs in a natural reciprocal pattern." She went on to say that with a neutral buoyancy device like the Wet Vest supporting core muscles, the child or adult could remain upright in the water. "Someone with hemiplegia will quickly discover that he has to use both arms and legs reciprocally to move forward in the water," she wrote. "If he relies on the old spastic pattern of depending upon the better-functioning side, he will just be able to go around in circles." [27]

It seemed that as a kid, I was in the water much of the time. From sunup to sundown, that's where I would be. Unfortunately, there was no such thing as a Wet Vest back when I was a tot, but life jackets would end up as a great substitute until I was strong enough and had developed sufficient coordination to swim. In the water I wasn't shy at all. Being timid was only for the landlubbers. Swimming underwater, I was like Jacques Cousteau. The characters in *Sea Hunt* and James Bond movies became my idols. I wanted to be just like them, always on some deepwater adventure, dreaming of scuba diving in crystal clear water. What a wonderful world that would be for a little kid with CP!

NEEDING AN EARLY "WIN" IN LIFE

Every young kid needs a win early in life to build confidence and trust in his or her abilities. For kids like me, it was even more crucial. But as my childhood life unfolded, I had subconsciously built the opposite; failure equates to an automatic flight response that unfortunately followed me for an exceedingly long time.

As an adult with CP and a master of several "wins" as of today, I highly encourage the moms and dads of kids with CP, or any disability, to discover what their kids' interests are, come alongside them, and do whatever it takes to help create that first authentic "win." This first win will build self-confidence that is so necessary for every other win to come. In my case, if I'd had a "win" around age five, doing, let's say, water-skiing, I might have built a healthy "fight response" instead of a "flight response," which was further reinforced time after time, shutting this little Leo down for years.

ICE-SKATING ON BUTTER

The reason we lived on Lake Austin is that my dad, Floyd McCreight, was (and still is) a well-known and respected American Water Ski Association competition water-skier.[28]

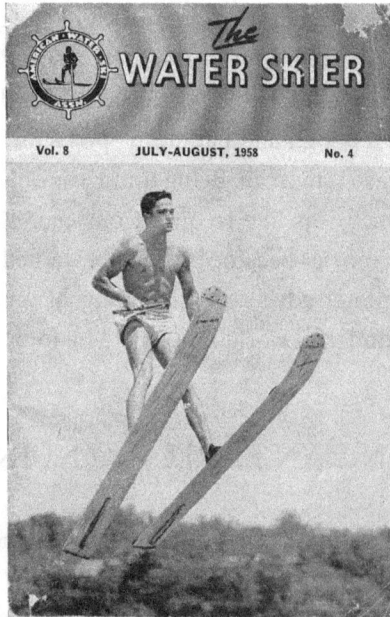

Floyd McCreight on the cover of The Water Skier magazine, 1958

Every summer, we would go to tournament after tournament across the country so he could compete in and judge competition water-skiing in trick, slalom, and jump. In 1972, Dad designed and built (alongside a general contractor) our lake house out of the rocky hillside on the lower end of Rivercrest Road, right on Lake Austin. We even had a ski jump right in front of our house.

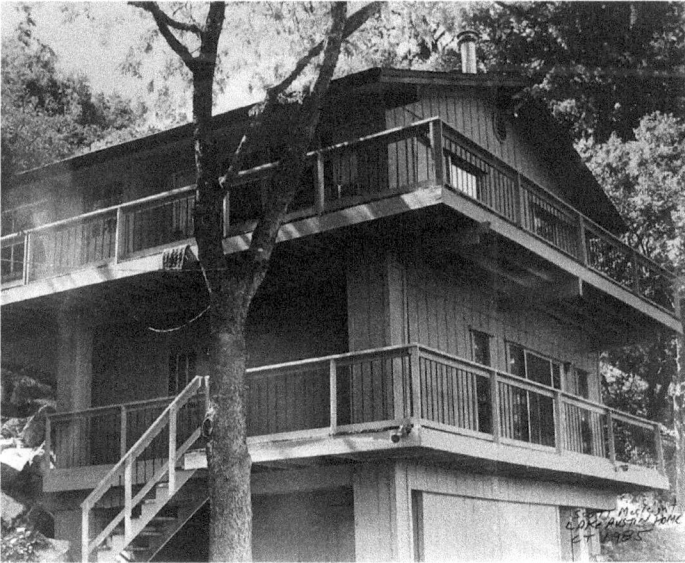

Our lake house out on Lake Austin in 1985

Our jump was on a rope pulley-type system, placing it in position for jumping and returning back to its moorings till next time. Watching skiing and jumping right in front of our house on those early mornings was exciting. Who else could boast that they had a ski jump in their front yard, much less a lake for a swimming pool? On early mornings, we would hop in our ski boat and go pick up Dad's ski buddies long before sunup, when the air was cold and thick with fog. Upon returning, we would untie the jump and hoist it into position, and we kids would scoop up water and keep the jump's waxed surface wet for the jumpers. These were the days before motorized pump systems were widely popular and inexpensive. We loved "volunteering" to do this job because we got to watch jumpers go over the jump from our protected platform under the high end of the ramp. This was an incredibly exciting experience. First we'd hear the ski boat get louder and louder as it approached from behind us. Then we'd hear the skis hitting the base of the ramp as the boat passed by on our right side. Then louder and closer, we would hear the skis approaching us, rumbling louder as the jump shook. We would sit on our platform, holding our ears and looking up. Up, up, and over we would hear the skier roar. Then we would see the skier leave the top of the ramp high above us, water would spray our faces, and the skier would fly over and land on the water in front of us. This was always a thrill. Not all landings were graceful, but they were always exciting for us kids. Deep down inside, I knew my dad wanted to raise his family to be competition water-skiers.

Before we built our house and lived on the lake, at around age four, I lived on Vallejo Street, in central Austin. Some of my earliest memories are of Dad water-skiing on Lake Austin. My sister, Karen, sat snug in her infant seat between my mother's legs as Mom drove our Hydrodyne competition ski boat. As evening approached and the sun was setting, we would make our way back up Bull Creek at what seemed to be an incredibly slow speed compared to the preceding activities, and we'd head to a secluded public boat ramp near an old hamburger restaurant (now known as the County Line). Then, with the smell of those hamburgers cooking nearby, Dad would back our old tan-colored Oldsmobile deep into the water with the tailpipe bubbling underneath. Remembering all those James Bond movies Dad took us to, I would try hard not to be in the back seat, or in the car at all, during this trailer submersion process, for reasons only secret agents knew about. After the boat was secured and fully wiped down, I got to lie down in the back seat as we drove home after sunset with our trusty boat in tow. We would drive up FM 2222, listening to the *Mystery Theater* broadcast on AM radio, which aired every Saturday and Sunday evening. When we arrived at home, Mom would run inside to turn on the radio so we would not miss any of the nail-biting story.

As we grew up, both my sister, Karen, and my stepbrother, Chris (my parents divorced when I was eleven years old, and my dad remarried Chris's mom, Linda), were singularly gifted at skiing, and I enjoyed watching everyone ski…from the safety of a ski boat. Due to my CP, my own water-skiing career would be short-lived. My dad tried everything in the book to get me up on water skis. Dad even hammered a board to the front of my little Kidder skis to keep my skinny legs together. Time after time, I would holler the command as loud as I could to the boat driver: "Hit it!" I'd feel the power of our trusted Ski Nautique roar to life, charging through the water, and then all hell would break loose. The kid with the frail body and big, oversized, bright-orange life jacket would crash in spectacular fashion. A feeling that I soon learned to dread from the moment I would get into the water from behind our boat.

"Houston, we have a problem!" Fall after fall, wipeout after wipeout, day after day. I did not like hitting the water at high speed, no matter what position I was in. I even tried to hang on to the ski rope as I fell, but then I was just dragged along for what seemed to be miles. I am proud to say that I did manage to get up on skis…eventually.

Being "graceful," however, was not part of this experience. Cerebral palsy continued to affect my balance and muscle coordination on my right side, so for me as a kid, getting up on water skis was like trying to ice-skate on skates made of butter while being pulled by a bull on steroids. Let's just say that I won several awards for the best fall on record—or would that be the *worst* fall? This further reinforced my sports theory: avoidance at all costs.

FAST CARS AND STICK SHIFTS

Driving a car seems like an ordinary task for most people. I was fortunate as a teenager in 1984 to begin my driving career with a sweet stick-shift, four-speed Datsun 280Z. It was an awesome car. Not a Nissan but a classic Datsun!

Sky blue, 1978, 2 + 2 model. I actually remember riding in that very same car as a kid, between the two back seats on that little hump, looking out the front window, holding on to the two handles above the side back windows as Dad drove fast around corners. Yes, those were the days before seat belts were required in the back seat.

Learning to drive can be rough for teenagers. It was *really* tough learning how to drive a stick shift, and even harder for me with CP. How was I to shift with my right hand, with little to no strength and grip? Confidence in what I could do as a teenager was foremost on the minds of a lot of people, including me. Even more complicated was shifting with my weak right hand, simultaneously pressing the velvet-touch clutch with my stronger left foot, while also steering (rack-and-pinion style) around corners with my left hand and applying just the right amount of gas with my CP right foot so I wouldn't stall or shotgun the car. What a complicated process with tight, complex timing!

This learned maneuver was ultimately a prelude to the beginnings of forced strengthening of my right hand and biceps in ways I would only fully realize when I started my transformation much later in life.

In those early days of 1984, I had been unable to firmly grip anything right-handed. Learning how to properly grip the stick shift while pressing a clutch constructed new pathways in my brain and neural system, something the doctors had said would likely never happen. The "experts" said that once brain damage occurs, it is *permanent*, and we all believed them because they were "the experts." These same experts also said that the brain is rigid and that once brain damage occurred, the brain would not repair itself.

I should have realized back then that driving that 280Z was proof that my brain was capable of neuroplastic behavior and that the brain does repair itself. My brain does adapt, and I was successfully adapting, growing new networks with every turn, every shift, each day. By driving that car, I was strengthening underused muscles in the process. This only occurred because my brain was actually changing neural "circuits," prompting my muscles to function. Sounds a lot like neuroplasticity in action to me.

UNLOCKING THE UNDERWATER WORLD

It was early spring, and my junior year of high school was about to start. One evening my mom showed me an article in our local newspaper, the *Westlake Picayune*. "Scuba Diving Lessons to Be Taught at Westlake High School" was the headline. As part of Westlake's continuing education program, they were going to offer classes for scuba diving. *Really? At my high school? Could I really do something like this? After all, I had CP. Surely they would not allow me to scuba dive with CP.* But I really wanted to learn how, and Mom knew it.

Mom asked me, "Scott, would you like to learn how to scuba dive?"

"Sure, Mom, sign me up!" I replied sarcastically, thinking to myself, *How am I going to pay for something like that? After all, scuba diving has to be very expensive.*

Before I knew it, Mom had signed me up and paid the eighty-five dollars for my Open Water scuba diving class at Scuba Point, a five-star PADI-certified provider, and just like that, I was in. I was going to learn how to scuba dive. Just like Jacques Cousteau, who was the first certified scuba diver in the world, I might add, and James Bond (the first stealth scuba diver). I, Scott McCreight, would join the elite masters of scuba diving. I would breathe underwater, and I would become a great diver. Now to convince my family doctor to let me do it...

As it turns out, my pediatrician had no issue at all with this concept. He figured I was already comfortable in the water, and there was nothing wrong with my ears or lungs. He signed off on my request.

The next two weeks waiting for the class to begin seemed like the longest of my entire life. I read up on everything I could find about scuba diving. There was no internet back in those days, so I had to actually go and hunt down information the old-fashioned way: I went to the library and researched this fascinating topic. I even found an old 1970s vintage *PADI Open Water Manual.*

And then my first night of scuba training finally arrived. I was excited and ready. I sat in the front row so I would not miss anything. My stepbrother, Chris, and several of my high school friends had also signed up. I think my excitement made it an easy sell for them. They say in marketing, "It's all about presentation and excitement." Well, let's just say that I sold lots of seats in that class.

The class would be structured in three parts: we would work through the book first at Westlake High in the evenings, then head to Scuba Point's heated indoor pool at the corner of FM 2222 and FM 620 (known to the locals as "Four Points"), then hit the open water at Windy Point on Lake Travis. Back then, there was only one Windy Point Park, and only scuba divers and their families ventured this far outside of Austin city limits. I couldn't wait to get into the water with all the scuba gear on. To learn how to breathe underwater! It was going to be so cool.

Scuba diving is very gear intensive. Equipment full of technology was everywhere, and I was ready to learn everything. Besides, James Bond had a lot of techie gear, and he must have had a ham radio or two around his spy shop somewhere (but I'm getting ahead of myself again).

Mitch Lambert and Tom McCoy were our PADI scuba diving instructors. They asked us to raise our hands if we didn't know how to swim. I thought this was a joke until I looked around and saw several hands raised. *How could anybody not know how to swim and want to scuba dive?* I thought. After all, I did learn how to swim before I walked. I was amazed at how many hands went up. I already had swimming mastered. This would be easier than I thought.

Bookwork was tough, but still, it was like I was made for the sport. I liked a sport! I never thought I would say that as a kid with CP. The lessons seemed easy. Even learning how to manipulate the dive tables and plan out dives seemed simple to me. Nitrogen absorption, maximum bottom time, no-decompression limits…it seemed intuitive. I found myself actually showing others in class how to work the tables on our predive simulations and working the math effortlessly. Dive equations came easy to me. It all made so much sense. Mitch even taught us how to survive a shark attack.

How many sharks could there be in Lake Travis? I thought. But I took notes with diligent detail. I learned how to hold the dive knife with the blade extended and that as the shark approached, you would swim over to your dive buddy, quickly stab, and swim away. The shark would be attracted to your buddy's blood…and you'd survive. Yes, I actually wrote that down in my notes. Odd, I thought, until I realized it was only a joke. We all wrote it down as if it was for extra credit or something.

Pool training was awesome. I learned how to clear my mask with no problem at all. All those hours at the lake house taught me how to do that as well as equalize my ears and more. I learned how to put scuba gear together, how to put my buoyancy compensator device—or BCD, later shortened to BC—on my tank, and how to properly put on all my gear and enter the water in several ways. I was even able to lift a standard eighty-cubic-foot scuba tank with my left hand, and that was the heaviest gear there was. Besides, everything in the water is essentially neutrally buoyant. Cerebral palsy didn't seem to affect me one bit underwater. Breathing was easy, and I had no fear at all. I had finally found the sport for me. It was the one sport I could master and would ultimately fall in love with.

When my dad found out I was actually interested in a sport, I think he was really excited. *His son was into a sport.* I can only imagine how proud he must have felt. He bought me my first Dacor XL scuba regulator and what was then called a dive computer (now known as a rudimentary bottom and surface interval timer) for Christmas. He even arranged for Dick Williamson—a friend of the family, fellow water-skier, and scuba divemaster—to dive with me.

Over the next several years, Dick and I would go out on scuba diving adventures in Lake Travis every weekend after I was certified. Dick became instrumental in building my self-confidence, increasing my proficiency, showing me the various underwater marvels, and deepening my understanding of what I could do with diving. He also introduced me to Austin's thriving scuba community and vast array of retail shops. There were around sixteen shops in the Greater Austin area back then. I did a lot of diving with Dick Williamson over the years. I learned new techniques, skills, and leadership abilities I never knew I had until scuba diving came along.

I seemed unaffected by CP underwater and felt like I was just like anybody else. It was a great feeling, being weightless, breathing air on life support called scuba, but best of all, *being normal.* In fact, I was doing something many normal people couldn't do or would never do. This was awesome. Sure, I had some problems reaching with my right hand, but underwater, it mostly didn't matter. Underwater you use your most powerful muscles, your legs, to propel you through the water. Your arms and hands are clasped in front of you, out of the way. Every movement underwater is slow and steady. The slow part I was used to; steady I was patiently working on. Dick Williamson and our diving experiences opened up a whole new world for me. More training! Technical dive training was soon to follow.

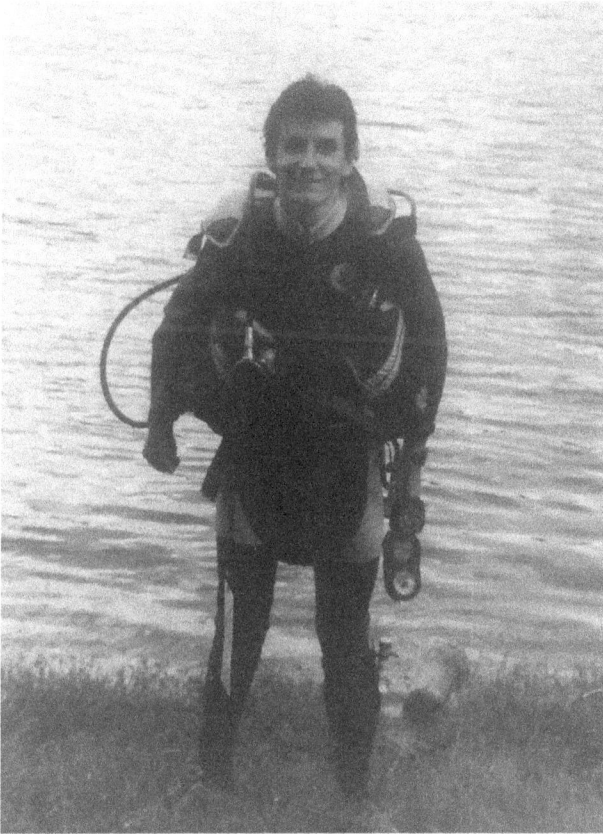

Me as a sixteen-year-old scuba diver

Leo Becomes a Techie

TECHNICAL TRAINING…I ATE IT UP WHEREVER I COULD FIND IT. Back a few years, I had started to become quite technical at everything I did; you could say I was a junior engineer at twelve years old. I loved tinkering with things. Always learning, I would try to figure out how everything worked, usually by taking things apart and putting them perfectly back together again. Well, except for that antique Underwood typewriter I persuaded my good family friend and at-one-time babysitter Kelly Osness to let us take apart one evening while she was looking after me. We both partook in the mechanical autopsy. Screws, gears, and parts were scattered about. We were never quite able to reassemble that Underwood the same as before, but we had so much fun attempting to.

I had gizmos and wires everywhere, like Dr. Emmett Brown from the *Back to the Future* movies. I even built my first ham radio while in junior high. By the time I was in high school, I would run around all over the neighborhood installing single sideband radios at my friends' houses so we could talk at all hours of the night. You could say that I had the whole neighborhood wirelessly wired. At the height of my junior communication company years, I must have had fifteen single sideband radios all over the West Lake Hills countryside, but that's a whole other story. All this technical learning and motivation I was eating up ended up being a catalyst for learning all the technical aspects of scuba diving.

A few years after my PADI Open Water scuba certification in 1986, I was once again back in Tom McCoy's advanced scuba diving class, where we were diving together on our first deepwater training dive at Lake Travis. By this time, I was no stranger to deep diving since Dick had taught me how to master these skills long before Tom's class, but deep down inside, I knew I needed to advance my qualifications if I ever hoped to officially climb the scuba certification ladder and be recognized for the achievements I was actively pursuing.

Tom and I had formed a special bond ever since my Open Water class at Westlake High School. He was impressed with my overall command of scuba diving over the years since then. He knew of my CP but never thought of it as a limitation. In fact, he told me years later that I inspired him to help others like me with neural-pathway conditions like CP. In his Advanced Open Water class, the other two students were young newlyweds, rushing through their training in preparation for a trip to Cabo San Lucas for their honeymoon. On our first deep dive, they both ran into trouble. Nitrogen narcosis can happen when a diver goes too deep. For some people, this makes you feel loopy; others "wig out." Then there are divers like me, who experience no ill effects at all. I was partnered with David, the newlywed, who was much bigger than me. We all started our descent into the cold, dark abyss. I followed my partner down.

Down, down we both went. A little faster than I would have preferred, but that was normal for the inexperienced diver I was partnered with. And I quickly recognized the early onset of "narcing out" in my dive partner. I tried to get his attention and calm him down, but he started to act irrationally. I looked at his gauges for signs of low air or deficiencies in his air supply. All were okay. He had plenty of air to breathe, and he was breathing fine. Suddenly, he started bolting for the surface from eighty feet down. I knew he was headed for trouble, possibly even the bends, if I did not act fast. Instincts instantly took over. I grabbed on to his weight belt and hung on tight to slow down his ascent. When we broke the surface, I ensured that he was positively buoyant and performed a quick medical check on him. He was stable, coherent, and calming down as I talked with him. He acted surprised and said he did not know what had come over him. His wife had also narced out; she had become loopy and wanted to descend deeper and deeper. Tom had to get her back topside. Her symptoms disappeared as well once she was on the surface and buoyant.

Later on, Tom and I debriefed from the day's events over barbecue at Smoky J's, at the corner of FM 2222 and FM 620 (the only place to eat for miles back then). "Nice rescue! Where did you learn how to do that?" he asked. "You should take my Rescue class next month." Yes, scuba diving instructors seem to always be selling. And I bought the whole scuba package from that point on.

My Rescue Diver class was extremely hard work. However, Tom commented that I had the fastest body recovery time of all his students in the class. This was due to all the members of our class helping me pull "the victim" (Tom) out of the water, so I could perform (simulated) CPR. At the time, I did not know if they were helping because I had CP and they "perceived" that I needed assistance or because I showed leadership and was able to enlist the whole team in the ongoing rescue. Perhaps both. In any case, Tom told us that in an emergency, it is all about teamwork. "And Scott was able to get all of you all to work together," he said. This quality was ultimately required to pass that class. No other team showed this skill before my turn.

After Rescue Diver certification, I branched out into technical dive training with certifications in scuba equipment repair and maintenance, advanced nitrox (O_2N), trimix (HeO_2N), and heliox (HeO_2) for very deep saturation diving, plus semi-closed rebreather (SCR), cavern and cave certifications, just to name a few.

MY FIRST DIVE MENTOR

While writing this book, I met with my scuba diving mentor, Dick Williamson, to rekindle old memories and stories for this book as well as his perceptions of coming alongside a young kid with CP and opening up my first "win." Among our many conversations over the years, Dick reminded me that he had known me my entire life. Dick is a family friend who recalls not only my scuba diving days but my life as a baby at those water-ski tournaments all the way to this day, a truly unique perspective. During our conversations, he helped me formulate this concept of a much-needed win in my life to build confidence that would lead to success at whatever I would do from that point on. We unpacked this concept and expanded upon the understanding that still, to this day, I avoid team sports and activities. Why is this? At the root, kids learn vital socializing skills from team sport activities. Team sports teach youngsters how to interplay and properly react to the various social and sports-related cues that ultimately develop healthy competitive team dynamics, known as team socialization. I did not learn this in a healthy sports-team type of dynamic. As a result, today I tend to "compete" with only myself and master a "sport" that is determined on one's own ability to master.

For instance, let's say, hypothetically, that my dad was not a champion water-skier but a champion-class scuba diver (if that even exists). Let's say my dad was a Jacques Cousteau–type of an example. Even though a kid of five years old cannot obtain his or her scuba certification at that age, I would have learned to dive by then because, after all, my dad was Cousteau, and no one would have told him no. In real life, I have known scuba diving prodigies that have learned to dive as small kids. So, in this scenario, I would have had my very first "win" becoming a scuba diver, which might've started instilling confidence in me at a younger age. I might have gone on from there, building confidence and social "team" skills and perhaps mastering other sports, such as snow skiing, for example, earlier in life. I would've gained the confidence to overcome my self-imposed limitations and fight for another win. This would've led to building even more confidence and driven me to go on to other future wins.

This hypothetical example that Dick and I constructed sparked a huge shift in my psychological understanding of cerebral palsy. Up to that point, I had been focusing mainly on the physical aspect of CP. However, there was an underlying current and more powerful mental component that I had not fully seen in constructing that "win" in young me—that of a brain–muscle alliance

(BMA) that was and is at play in all of us. These new psychological constructs presented in my various conversations with Dick really sparked a renewed interest in positively altering early childhood development patterns by adding "wins" for kids with cerebral palsy.

When you give hope to a young kid with CP and establish their first win, the consequent mental drive will ultimately spark a forest fire of successes way beyond just that of the physical aspect of development. I wanted to lead others in this brain–muscle alliance. I wanted to help build success in others—not only by way of neuromuscular plasticity but also ultimately in developing self-confidence for success.

Leo Begins to Question Destiny

AFTER HIGH SCHOOL, WHILE MY FEW CLOSE FRIENDS WERE FINISHING up college entrance exams and mounds of paperwork, I found myself questioning where I was really supposed to be headed in life. Since I had learned over and over again that I was not smart enough to attend college, and my parents were not encouraging me to go to college like other kids' parents were, what was a kid with CP to do after high school? Somewhere along the way, I thought that attending a nationally known high-tech trade school might be my answer, working toward a two-year associate's degree. I could learn a trade and perhaps open a VCR repair shop or something similar. Okay, so how would I get into a school like that? My high school transcript and a lot of bucks later, there I was in the classroom, learning basic electronics or, as they say, electrical engineering technology (EET).

It was fun and exciting. Learning electronic theory—like Ohm's law, Moore's law, RLC circuit analysis, resonant circuit design, and how voltage and current were related—was surprisingly easy for me. I learned and built analog circuits like RC ladders and digital circuits such as AND gates, NAND gates, and OR gates out of basic components. How these circuits manipulated voltage and current was fascinating. Surprisingly, this learning environment boosted my confidence and gave me a fundamental understanding about the childhood electronics projects I had done many years ago. After all, I had built my first amateur radio at eleven years old. But up to this point, I had not fully grasped the concepts of how it all worked.

In tech school, I was always on the dean's list with a 4.0. I was eating this stuff up with a big-boy fork. By my second year, I was going to school in the morning, doing homework in the afternoon, sleeping early evenings, then working a full-time night shift for Motorola off of West William Cannon in Oak Hill, a semiconductor manufacturing company in Austin, Texas, now known as NXP.

I thought this job would lead to a good career, growth, and advancement after my graduation. Work, school, homework, sleep…then start all over again— but this began to wear thin. I started to notice an inner tug deep within my spirit, whispering to me: *You are not where you need to be. There is more out there that you need to experience. You are meant for greater things to come.*

I noticed that all of my friends from high school were off at university, studying, partying in their dorms, and experiencing life, "real" life. I felt that I was missing out on those experiences. Those were the dreams I wanted for myself. Nothing but work, trade school, sleep…it all became bland and unfulfilling. I also started getting little nudges at work, more whispers. Things like seeing "older" workers doing the same job for twenty years or more, with little or no passion. *You are meant for much, much more, Scott.* I was only nineteen years old, and I couldn't see myself still doing this when I was forty. The more I tried to ignore the nudges, the more depression started to sink in. The "twisted sisters," as I called them—better known as depression and anxiety—were rearing their ugly heads in my life, and I was ripe and unprotected from their talons. As time progressed, the whispers grew louder and louder.

At work, I served on my first board, the Motorola QCB, which stood for quality control board. In hindsight, this was my first glimpse into industrial system engineering practices, but more on that later. Motorola had coined the concept of Six Sigma quality for manufacturing a few years earlier, and we thrived on it on the factory floor. It was the QCB that ignited a spark in me that would ultimately lead me on a whole new trajectory. I started to listen to that whisper. I wanted more; I wanted to experience what *normal* kids were doing. I wanted to go to college.

THE HIGHWAY OF DESTINY

By March 1987, destiny grabbed hold of me and shook me up quite a bit. Up to this point in my life, I had come to think of destiny as a "weak force," like gravity. A force that seems weak but has a very strong, slow pull over time. I envisioned myself on an eight-lane highway heading north. Destiny was that road north. The various lanes represented choices of what I could do in life, while still heading north. What I sensed deep within my core was that I was no longer on this highway heading north but on a tiny, all but forgotten road parallel to the highway. I was still heading north, but the road was becoming bumpier and curvier as I strayed from the highway—the road was leading me farther away. I had to get back onto that highway. Once there, I had to speed up, or I would miss my destination altogether. I would miss out on something amazing.

But how? What did this all mean in the "real world" I was living in? How could I translate the metaphors into something real? More whispers would soon come, soft whispers: *Scott, you must attempt. You must go to college. You are destined for more.* I kept sensing and beginning to listen to that spirit within me. I needed to go to college.

CLIMBING THE COLLEGE MOUNTAIN

There were several people I still had to convince about my plan for going to college—most of all myself. There was another voice I had listened to before, the loud one. The one that told me so many times that I was not smart enough, that I was not college material. After all, the proof was clear. My SAT and ACT scores from Westlake High School were low, due to not caring about those tests. I was not going to college, so why try? How could I refute this evidence? I also had to convince my parents. "Oh, hi, Mom and Dad. I think I now want to go to school at a university." How would that go over? And then there were the colleges themselves. How would I get in? Why would they want to accept a kid with CP and low test scores into their university? It all seemed like a tall, insurmountable mountain to climb.

Still, that gentle spirit within me was turning up the volume. Or was I just beginning to listen? Clarity. I was ready to start listening. The feeling that I must try, that I must go to college, was stronger than ever. I was at the bottom of a pit, and all I could do was stop digging and just look up.

Starting at the bottom meant quitting my job and career lifeline at Motorola. Surprisingly, doing this was both liberating and gratifying. My second step was to enroll in classes at my local community college to see if I could handle a college-level class while continuing to go to trade school in the mornings.

That first semester at Austin Community College, I took two courses, English and history. Learning to study came easier than it did for most students in community college because I was already doing it in my morning trade school program. My mom, an English teacher by vocation, was not only happy to see me try out college but once again ended up being my greatest advocate. She would make sure I did my assignments and would look over my shoulder to make sure I was spelling words correctly in all my essays. She was part mom, part schoolteacher, but always supportive of my drive and desire to succeed. The classes were exciting as well. With the drive to "return to that highway" burning hot inside and the fortitude and determination to succeed, I was starting to feel like my bumpy, curvy road was turning toward that high-way. By the end of that first semester, I received my first college report card and made straight As in both classes along with remaining on the dean's list in my trade school program. But would I be able to continue? Doubts tried to creep in; they yelled and screamed at me. Second semester came and went with History 2 and English Composition. Again, Mom was there looking over my shoulder, but it was I who penned every word, studied every chapter, and mastered every exam. Again, I would wait by the mailbox for my report card to arrive. Another series of straight As served as a reward for my effort and determination.

My next step was to find a school and degree plan and get everything I needed ready to apply. An unexpected bonus came my way: now that I had college credit from my community college work, I no longer had to rely on my low SAT or ACT scores I would just need to supply my college transcript and my high school diploma and grades.

The University of Texas was my next step. I decided to take a class at UT as a transient student, which means I was taking classes without a degree plan or guarantee of getting into a school under the university in the future. As it turned out, I also did well at UT, gradewise, but the campus and the student-to-teacher ratio and learning structure were not as conducive to learning as I'd hoped—or required.

In the days before the internet, I had to research schools the old-fashioned way. I called, wrote, and visited a few other schools around Texas to see their campuses and research their degree programs. I decided to apply to Texas Tech University, located in a sleepy little town known as Lubbock, as far from Austin as one can get and still be in Texas. I planned to study engineering, and the school seemed perfect. After applying and waiting what seemed like an eternity, I was conditionally accepted on the conditions that I graduate with my EET associate's degree and my junior college grades remained above a 3.2 GPA.

That Christmas, I was going to fly out to San Diego to spend the holiday with Dad and my stepmother, Linda, and present them with my plan…a plan that might give my dad a heart attack, great joy, or perhaps both. My plan was to graduate from my technical school and transfer into Texas Tech University to become an engineer. My dad, a retired commander in the Navy, had gone to the University of Texas and earned both an undergraduate degree in mechanical engineering and a master's in aerospace engineering. I think deep down inside, he hoped his son would become an engineer too.

My proposal to Dad was all prepared, and my college grades and past performance entered as evidence. I packed the 1988 *Texas Tech University Handbook*, with the electrical engineering program highlighted, dog-eared, and memorized. I rehearsed my talking points and refined and practiced them with Mom. It would be the hardest sell in all of history: to convince Dad that his son, CP or not, was going to go to college and become an engineer. But I thought I was ready.

I was extremely nervous about presenting my plan to my father, retired Commander McCreight. I was worried that he would not like my plan and he would say no. After all, he had just spent a lot of money to put me through trade school, and now I wanted to attempt college?

After arriving in Del Mar, a San Diego suburb out in Southern California, it took three days before I mustered the nerve to approach this delicate, course-altering moment. Then the time came, the mood was right, and the conditions were ripe for bearing fruit. I approached Dad that evening and asked to speak with him for a few minutes.

"Dad, can I talk with you a moment or two?" I squeaked out after clearing my throat a couple of times. *Was it getting hot in here?* I thought.

Dad and I went into his dark den, and I proceeded to lay out my proposal and show him my transcripts and research. I conveyed my passion and drive to return to school and earn a bachelor of science degree in electrical engineering. My head was spinning. I could hear my heart beating wildly in my ears, and my body was shaking inside, but I forged on and projected confidence and courage throughout this presentation.

He stood there, silently looking over the material, studying it. He then sat down to fully take in the magnitude of this venture his son was proposing. After what seemed like an eternity of silence, he responded. "You know, I met your mom at Texas Tech," he said. "You want to study to become an engineer? That's a great idea."

I was stunned. This was not the reaction I expected.

Then I thought I might faint, so I quickly sat down on the couch next to him. We had to hash out the details, but he was "a go" with my plan. I think he must have felt proud that his son was going to follow in his footsteps. Military officers are trained never to show emotion to their men, but I could see it in his eyes that night.

I ended up graduating early from my associate's degree program with straight As and finishing up my UT and ACC classes way above the required 3.2 GPA in order to make the beginning of the 1988 fall semester at Texas Tech—and start my new life. I would live in a dorm, have a roommate, and study engineering. I'd finally get to experience what my friends had been telling me about a few years back. Leo was going to university! I was once again back on the highway of destiny.

College Life for Leo

FOR MOST KIDS WHO GO OFF TO COLLEGE, IT'S A TIME OF GREAT change and growth. What you learn outside the classroom is often more important, intense, and life-changing than what you learn inside the classroom. College is all about growing up and learning how to deal with life. For me, this would be doubly so. I fought long and hard to be among the kids who now call the Texas Tech University campus home. I had made it! I was in college, starting life in college as a regular student. I would no longer be treated like a shy, introverted kid with CP. I was about to experience everything a *normal* college student would experience—no longer letting CP hold me back. Yep, it felt great. I would be considered normal here.

DORM LIFE

My first semester at Texas Tech was fun and exciting. It was filled with so much change that I wanted to remember everything. I wanted to experience everything that a college student would experience...well, almost everything. I was a few years older than most students, so I had more "common sense" than some of my new college pals. I decided to start journaling at this point in my life because I knew there was about to be a radical shift in my learning and growth, and I wanted to capture and process everything. After all, the highway I was now traveling down seemed to be growing more lanes to choose from, and I wanted to capture as much of this growth as I could.

Socially, college life was off to a great start as well. Bledsoe Hall, room 145, would be my home for at least the next year. This would be my first dorm room. It took me a full two days until I even met my roommate. John Frazier was a sophomore and computer science undergrad who worked for the university. He was cool. He was on the residence halls association (RHA) and worked in the Bledsoe office. We hung out together when he was not working or in class. John was taking eighteen hours that semester, which meant he was often busy. His girlfriend, Amanda, lived across campus at Gates Hall, so we tended to hang around there much of the time. I still felt shy and introverted around girls due to years of low self-confidence and the perceived difficulties around my CP.

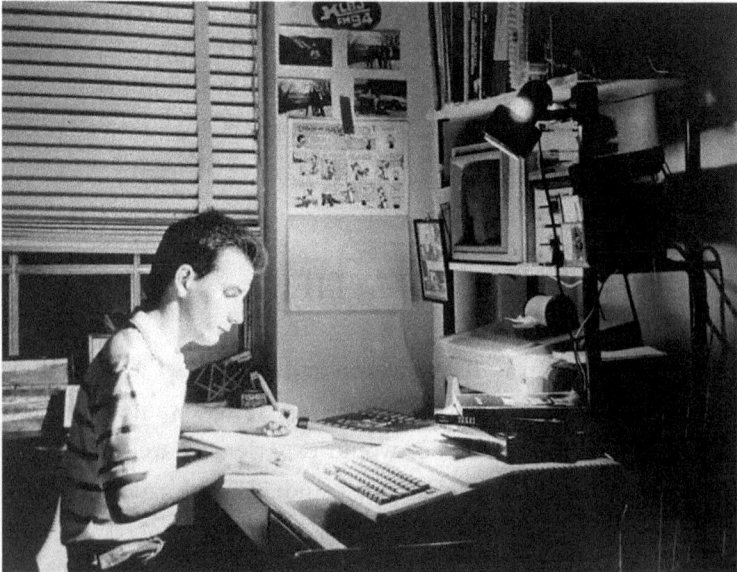

In Bledsoe Hall dorm, 1988

MEETING LIFELONG FRIENDS

I took a full load of classes my first semester; most were prerequisites for my electrical engineering major. Chemistry class was taught by a noticeably young PhD, Dr. Bruce R. Whittlesey. He taught his class in a semicircular lecture room with seats on risers. The room was dark, small, and cramped. He looked and acted so much like us that he told us to call him Bruce. In fact, he insisted. One early morning in class, he began lecturing about some exciting chemistry topic that escapes me now, when in runs this skinny kid, late and in a rush. Upon finding no open seats except for right in front of Bruce, he sat quickly—and noisily, I might add. Bruce looked at him and paused long enough to stifle a smile. Bruce began his lecture once again, only to be interrupted by this same guy attempting to open a soda can he'd brought to class. What happened next still, to this day, makes me laugh. The guy tapped the lid in rapid succession, "tap, tap, tap," before pulling the tab to open the can. All of a sudden, the can started to explode all over the place. It sprayed everywhere, in what could be described as a volcano ejecting pyroclastic streams of soda in high arches. This phenomenon was akin to mixing Mentos and Diet Coke, producing a violent reaction in slow motion—so much so that this guy picked up his backpack, exploding soda and all, and ran out the same door he had just come in. Bruce stopped lecturing, watched the kid's hasty departure, and chuckled. "Soda-catalyzed eruption reaction in action," he said. Then he laughed and continued with his lecture.

"What a dork!" I remember saying to the guy next to me. "Glad I'm not that kid." And the kid never came in late again.

To my surprise, a week or so later, I ran into this guy in Bledsoe. Damon Cox lived upstairs in room 321 and was an electrical engineering student like me. We hit it off and became good friends. Guess you really should not judge a book by its cover—ever! Damon later told me that he had overslept that fateful day and was in a rush to get to chemistry. He had grabbed a soda from his dorm fridge and run to class. He had only realized the can was partially frozen when he opened it, and the forceful spray was a result of pressure applied to a frozen mass up near the top. I could not help but laugh again upon telling Damon about Bruce's reaction. This exploding Coke can, and some ironic chemistry, started a friendship that we still enjoy to this day. Damon often says that I never cease to amaze him with my determination and dedication. As he puts it, "Scott is very hardworking and takes great pride in everything that he does."

Not all friendships start out with exploding ordnance, but they often end up that way. Zachary Joe Zachary is such a friend. I met Joe, or Z^2 as we called him on account of his name, in Bledsoe. Joe lived on the other end of the dorm and was a cool guy to hang with. We went out to clubs together to listen to music, drink, and have a good time. When Joe graduated that next year, he entered the Army and was stationed in Iraq during Operation Desert Shield and Operation Desert Storm. I sent him letters every so often and even sent him more than five hundred magazines and other "field supplies" for him and his Army buddies to read. Joe would receive these letters and packages from Texas Tech while in the field with live rounds going off all around him. He told me that my packages really cheered everyone up out in the field. After Desert Storm, Joe came back to Texas Tech for grad school my senior year. We picked right up as if nothing had separated us. Some of the gang had filtered in and out, but we were still best buds. He would often comment to me that I would accomplish more than most normal people would ever be able to do. Joe did not see me as someone with CP but simply as a cool college student.

James is another friend with whom I've held a lifelong bond. I met James Crutchfield in Bledsoe as well. He was into computers and Army stuff. I thought this was a weird combination, but I had seen a lot of weird combinations in college. James and I also hit it off. He grew up near Houston and frequented the Austin area as a kid. Many of his stories of growing up seemed remarkably familiar to me, but I was unable to put my finger on *why*. He told odd stories of family reunions and cousins he had in the Austin area. I later learned that one of his cousins was one of my best friends growing up at Eanes. I recognized his stories of family reunions out on their family farm because I must have attended one or two of these get-togethers as a guest of his cousin, Matt Kocks, when we were young. God has a funny way of bringing people together. Like Joe, James has never seen me as someone incapable of doing things because of CP. He recognizes that CP has accelerated the determination in me to do the things that I have now mastered.

ACADEMIC CHALLENGES WITH CP

Academically, my first semester was off to a rocky start. By mid-semester, I was failing my trigonometry class. Although I invested massive hours studying, I still failed tests. And as a result, it pulled my other classes down. I vividly remember calling home one evening and talking with Mom. How could I be doing badly in trig as an engineering student? Would this be the end? Was I going to fail out my very first semester of college? As usual, Mom compassionately listened, and her teacher instinct kicked into high gear. She suggested I work smarter, not harder. She researched and talked with a few folks, including Barbara Watt (from earlier in this book). Barbara suggested I call the assistant dean of students and ask for assistance. The very next day, I scheduled an appointment and nervously went to visit Trudy Potite. During our meeting, Trudy explained that the Americans with Disabilities Act (ADA) of 1990 was set up to help kids like me, kids with CP. According to the ADA National Network:

> The ADA is a civil rights law that prohibits discrimination against individuals with disabilities in all areas of public life, including jobs, schools, and transportation, as well as all public places and private places that are open to the general public. The purpose of this law is to make sure that people with disabilities have the same rights and opportunities as everyone else. The ADA gives civil rights protections to individuals with disabilities similar to those provided to individuals on the basis of race, color, sex, national origin, age, and religion.[29]

What struck me the most about Trudy was her compassion to my cause because, like me, she was also disabled. We could relate to each other, and that gave me great comfort in my struggle. She helped me to understand that reasonable accommodations had to be provided and extended and that I would first need to prove my disability since I had not declared one upon entering school. She told me I would need my disability record on file with the university before we could work on a formal solution. However, she also said she would work on getting provisional approval before my paperwork came in from the State of Texas Health and Human Services Commission, or HHSC (known as the Texas Rehabilitation Commission [TRC] back in 1988).

Paperwork? What paperwork would this be? And what was this TRC? I wondered.

This was way before the days of the internet or email, so I had to call HHSC and ask what the TRC was. I asked whom I could talk with about my records. The TRC keeps files of everyone in the state who has a rehabilitation record, from the time of their diagnosis, including accommodations in primary school, to any required records throughout high school. TRC must have kept these records in a vault somewhere because many phone calls later, I finally found the right person to ask for a copy of my original diagnosis and other related paperwork to be sent to Texas Tech. Most were from a case file they had kept on me from my early days at the Austin CP Center and upon entering elementary school. I never knew records like this even existed. These records were of great importance. I later found out that this paperwork and assistance from the assistant dean's office would have made applying and acceptance into Texas Tech less painful, but that was water under the bridge.

Trudy suggested that I take all my math exams in their monitored testing center and said that I would be granted "time and a half" allowances for completing all assigned tests. Then the tests would be sent back to the professor for grading and processing. She also set up some tests to evaluate what else, if anything, would be of assistance for me.

That first phone call and related chain of events were the difference between night and day for me. From certain failure to hope for success, this was a true unforeseen blessing. My grade point average rose to a 3.56 by the end of my first semester. This time and a half on math exams was all I needed to figure out how to process these mathematical concepts that were giving me so much trouble. "You should not be ashamed of needing these services," Trudy said. "After all, Einstein suffered from the same thing in math that you have. You just need to reorient the way you comprehend these complex mathematical concepts."

Leo Becomes an Amateur Radio Operator

WE ALL HAVE DREAMS AND HOPES AS KIDS. JUST LIKE BECOMING A certified scuba diver, I also very much hoped that I would someday become a General class ham radio operator. People who talk and operate amateur radios are known as ham radio operators. I'm not quite sure where the term *ham* came from. Was it a shortened word used for amateur? Or do these folks just like to "ham it up" by practicing their craft? Nevertheless, this group of people would set up radio equipment and talk to other ham operators all over the world using special radio frequencies set aside for noncommercial purposes: for teaching, disaster relief, and all sorts of hobby-related activities.

Ever since I was a young boy, I had been fascinated with communications and how people would use radios and antennas to spread messages and communicate all over the world. I had dreamed of being one of these ham radio people and, as I mentioned earlier, had even built my first radio at age eleven.

One of my fondest memories occurred while sitting at the dining room table of our lake house as a preteen. Just as in Netflix's *Stranger Things*, I had a pair of TRC-214, three-channel, crystal-controlled Radio Shack walkie-talkies—complete with their covers removed, inner workings and electronic components and power cells out on the table for full autopsy. As Dad diagrammed a radio system and how it worked, I was drawn deeply into this magical world. He wrote out electrical circuits and math that looked complicated. I was intrigued...I was fascinated at how electricity could be harnessed to do this, and I wanted to know more! Fast-forward to Texas Tech, and I was well into my electrical engineering coursework. But still, I wanted to be a ham radio operator.

David W. Duke, a skinny, spunky, blond-haired kid and fellow resident of Bledsoe Hall, was always walking down the halls with this cool-looking radio on his belt. Everyone called him "Hamster," a weird but foretelling name. His radio was a much smaller version of that old Radio Shack walkie-talkie I had disemboweled many years ago. It was a Kenwood TH-25AT, a similar radio model to the one Bruce Willis would sport in the movie *Die Hard 2* later that same year. However, this one was the two-meter version. Bruce had the TH-45AT (seventy-centimeter version), after all. Bruce was out in Los Angeles, California, where seventy-centimeter radios must have been more popular, I thought. David showed me not only this tiny radio but also that he was a licensed ham radio operator, hence his nickname, "Hamster." His call sign was KB5IZO (now known as KM5YQ), and he soon became my ham radio Elmer. *Elmer* is a term given to those who help mentor others with this incredibly vast hobby.

I must admit, the irony of an eighteen-year-old kid sitting down with a twenty-one-year-old EE student was not lost on me. He had moxie and a passion for radio like I did—I was fully humbled and committed to his tutoring. He soon pulled out this big book called the *ARRL Handbook*, a thick hardcover book filled with what seemed like a cornucopia of radio theory knowledge. We spent hours sitting in the hallways of Bledsoe outside of room 322, which I now called home, studying all sorts of radio theory. He said that to get a Novice class radio license, I would need to learn Morse code at five words per minute and understand some basic radio theory. However, to be able to operate one of these radios, he said as he held up that Kenwood Handie-Talkie (HT), I would need to take another theory test to receive a Technician class license. I was nervous, but I was all in. To administer the test, David would set up two General class operators, called VEs or volunteer examiners, when the time came. I studied theory with David and practiced receiving Morse code every free moment I had. After all, I had a dream and a destiny to fulfill. My prize would be my very own license and an HT like David had.

The fall semester was soon upon us, and it was time to take my exam. I arrived early that day, before semester classes were to start, and headed up to the second floor of the psychology building at Texas Tech University. This was where I would take my Novice code exam and theory. Looking back at this experience today, it was fitting that my test was held in the windowless building at Tech known as "the psychology building," where all sorts of strange and mysterious human and animal experiments took place. Was I taking part in one of them? I narrowly passed the code portion by the skin of my ear because I was so nervous. However, I made a 100 percent on my written exam after my relief from passing the code test. I was victorious. I patiently waited six weeks to the day as my FCC Form 610 was processed at the FCC headquarters and a license was generated and issued in my name. I officially became KB5LRF and soon took my Technician theory exam and was ready for my very own HT.

Paying it forward and rooting for the underdog became my unofficial motto beginning at Texas Tech. In fact, rooting for the underdog is still my motto to this day. I have even been called a sheepdog by my military friends because of this philosophy. I wanted to give back to others as I had been so given, if not give even more. In part, I wanted to become a VE, or Volunteer Examiner, while I was at Texas Tech, to help give to others that which others had given to me. I ended up spending three years as a VE for Lubbock's ham community, sporting my very own HT on my belt (Yeasu FT-470). I also helped create and run a ham radio club called the Tech Amateur Radio Society under Gerald Grant, our advisor, call sign WB5R. I ended up climbing all the way up the ham radio ladder with generous help from the Orange County RACES Club and Gordon West (WB6NOA) through the Advanced class certification process and very shortly after to Amateur Extra. I was then issued the call sign N5ZL—all while attending Texas Tech.

Looking back, all I had really wanted as a kid was to be a General class ham radio operator, a class I actually skipped right over to climb to the very top with demonstrated proficiency of well over twenty words per minute (WPM) Morse code and five radio theory tests under my belt (my highest speed was thirty-two WPM). Hope is indeed powerful.

Leo Unknowingly Joins a Fraternity

How does one unknowingly join a fraternity? During my junior year at Texas Tech, I found myself in this unlikely predicament. Joining a fraternity was an experience I thought I would never be interested in, or rather want to experience, or even be accepted as a candidate. After all, I was turning into an engineer geek and still felt socially inept. Jim Hall, an old friend from Austin, decided to transfer to Texas Tech and wanted to go through what is called Interfraternity Council Rush—a formal structured process in which one visits several fraternities to see how you both like each other. I envisioned this process like a cross between interviewing and speed dating rolled into one big series of parties.

I wanted no part of this rush stuff, but I did join Jim for a couple of parties at the Sigma Tau Gamma house right off Broadway, down from campus. It was before classes started and I had just passed my amateur radio exam to become a licensed ham radio operator. I wanted to party a little bit to celebrate one of my first lifelong goals that I had successfully achieved. I did and had a fantastic time.

After my intense amateur radio exam, I was ready to blow off some steam before getting ready for class, while catching up with my old friend from Austin over beers. This seemed like a cool thing to do. Did I mention that the beer was free? That next week, I received a card under my dorm door. I had been extended a formal bid to join the Kappa pledge class of Sigma Tau Gamma. *What was this invitation? What was a bid?* I had achieved something I was not even attempting to go after!

Could a guy with CP be part of a fraternity? And what were the odds of this without even trying out for the part? I was excited and nervous all at the same time. I ended up joining Sigma Tau Gamma and went through the pledge routine mostly unscathed. After all, I was an older pledge who had a wee bit more sense not to fall for the ol' pranks of snipe hunts, kidnappings, or penny-the-door-shut routines. I met and got to know several young men who held some of the same values and high standards I had learned and practiced over the years.

My Big Brother, Curt Burlbaw, helped me become an *active* and kept me out of too much trouble. As an *active*, I had three Little Brothers over the years—Will, Scott, and Bryan. Bryan Cotton was my last Little Brother. I am so proud of all my Little Brothers for not only putting up with me as a Big Brother but also pledge-ship and becoming active members. Since Bryan was my last Little Brother, he had to go through the most "hell" before becoming an active; he had to endure a whole lot of nasty stuff that Sigma Tau Gamma was going through in those final days. I even offered him the opportunity to de-pledge before he became an active brother since nationals were wanting to shut down our colony for various reasons, and we thought it was best to shield him from it all—he declined and stood by my side to the very last chapter meeting before we closed the doors in the fall of 1992. I appreciated all the trust he had in me and that he wanted to finish the race by my side. Nobody considered me unable or unworthy of brotherhood due to CP, especially Bryan.

RUNNING 101

Unless you're an athlete on scholarship, physical fitness in college is not typically something anybody actively thinks about at this point in life. I was comped out of all my physical fitness elective credits due to my expansive scuba diving experiences and various certifications, so I was not required to attend any sports-related classes; thank God for small miracles. Again, something that my younger days drilled into me: I do not do competition sports well. And I was not about to tempt fate with this in college. However, I did take up jogging around the campus my first year. In those days at Texas Tech, there was an uneven, rocky, and dusty five-mile cowpath jogging trail around the main campus. I started running this path with Edwin (Winn) Whiting, one of my childhood friends who had encouraged me for many years. Winn was more in shape than I was, and he really wanted to be a Marine from his early days as a child. Winn pushed me a little farther and harder than I, with my thin legs and poor muscle tone on my right side, would have liked. I also didn't understand what the concept of running at pace was all about. All I knew was how to sprint or how to fast-walk, but everything in between was more like a sprint-fast-walk routine with a very tall, long-legged guy like Winn. To keep up with him, I seemed to always be at a sprint. Those were the days before heart rate monitors and high-tech watches, so there was no way of determining biofeedback mechanisms like heart rate, breathing rate, and fatigue in real time. My running was more like a full-out sprint, tired-out walk, sprint again, repeat. My gait was not normal due to my right leg spasticity and lack of foot strength. But I did my best. Joe Zachary even commented that I had a lot of determination to "run the loop" with Winn. This was something he himself wished he could have done back then. Joe ended up joining the Army years later and learned what physical training was really about. To this day, however, Joe still commends me for being able to keep up with Winn on that cowpath running trail.

Other than running around the campus or getting out on a five-story wall to teach rappelling to a few adventurous friends—learning rope work and practicing safety procedures—I spent most of my time in the library exercising my brain instead. After all, I was going to be an engineer, and to do that, I had to pass my classes, learn to "play the game," and graduate. I found that studying was a nice retreat from some of the socially awkward situations I was not good at dealing with. Nothing was going to get in the way of me becoming an engineer, but having some fun and living in the dorms were some of the most exciting times of my life...so far.

SNOW SKIING WITH CP

Snow skiing, for most people, is a sport that, once learned, will be enjoyable for years to come. However, for folks with diplegia or hemiplegia cerebral palsy, snow skiing is all *but* fun and, for some, seems to be just a dream. My first experience with snow skiing was in 1974, at the early age of seven in Vail, Colorado. Kiddo ski school was not fun for me due to my lack of control going downhill and being a shy kiddo. In those days, kids did not wear helmets. I should have worn one. Due to a lack of ability to plow or cut, I couldn't control my speed. While most kids were doing nice, slow, gentle "S-curves" down the mountain, I was the kid who put the two straight lines right down the center of the dollar sign symbol, every time, without fail. The instructors tried to teach me, but I still cut for the bottom as fast as my tiny skis would take me. Like water-skiing, snow skiing was not for me.

This would all change in the winter of 1992 at the age of twenty-five.

SKIING IN A WHOLE NEW LIGHT

During the Christmas break of 1992, I spent time on a vacation with my father, stepmother, and stepbrother, Chris. We packed up the car and headed to the Mammoth Lakes ski resort, 450 miles north of San Diego. When we arrived, there was close to three and a half feet of snow on the ground at our lodge. This Texas boy had not seen this much snow since I was seven years old.

We went to get measured for ski equipment and to get ready to hit the slopes the next day. I was feeling uneasy. I still vividly remembered my last ski adventure from 1974, and I was not wanting to repeat this failure. I was grateful that my dad enrolled me in ski lessons.

December 26 was the first day of ski school. Fear can be a powerful motivator. Fear of the unknown or of memories and/or actions can be even more motivating. To add to this uneasiness, I don't like to be in crowds, and it sure seemed crowded out there on the slopes. I felt nervous and unsure of myself and what I was about to do over the next several days. However, as the first day wore on, I was so busy practicing my newly learned techniques from ski school that I did not notice the crowds at all, and my fear slowly gave way to confidence from achievements on the slopes. Ski school, this time, turned out to be a great experience, highly recommended for those of us with "fear issues."

Mike was my A-School ski instructor, and our class consisted of twelve people, ranging in ages from seventeen to thirty-five. I learned all sorts of stuff a new skier needs to master to survive the slopes. Like how to stop by using the snowplow and side turn, how to sidestep, and even the all-popular how to turn your skis around while standing in place (my favorite yoga torture move). We even learned to recover from various types of falls (I was already an expert at this part). And we learned how to get up using poles and how to remount skis in deep snow. After lunch, we headed down our first "beginner trail," appropriately named Sesame Street West. We made four runs down this trail; however, I only accomplished three because I had trouble making the snowplow with my right leg and foot, and I did not want to hold up the group any longer than I already had. Frankly, at this point, I just wanted to quit and give up. However, Mike was persistent, helpful, and patient with my lack of control and "ability" and kept encouraging me to continue learning. Due to CP affecting my right leg and foot and contributing to poor muscle tone, I had great difficulty performing the snowplow correctly with the right side of my body. As a result of this imbalance, I would sharply turn to my left side.

Mike went way above and beyond what an instructor typically does. He actually skied down backwards in front of me while holding his ski pole horizontally out in front of his body so that I could grab onto it; this helped to slow me down and keep my pace steady. He also gave me a lot of pointers along the way. I hoped that his pointers would eventually help me master the snowplow on my own. Otherwise it was going to be a miserable experience going down every slope with Mike in front of me.

The next morning, I went on to B-School. Brent Allen was my instructor. He had been skiing for twenty-one years and instructing for most of that time. There were eleven others in my class. Brent was aware of my problem performing the snowplow turn from the previous day, even before I could mention it. He said he had a solution to this problem that would most likely help my weak right side form a perfect snowplow. I was intrigued.

He then reached into his coat pocket and pulled out what looked like a little colorful rubber hose. As he attached this device to the tips of my skis, he told me it was called an Edgie Wedgie.[30] "This should do the trick," he said. It was basically a piece of surgical tubing with two clamps on each end, designed to form a snowplow. As I would spread my legs, my larger and stronger abductor muscle group (located on the lateral side of the thigh) would cause my legs to spread apart. The resistance of the tubing would cause my ski tips to remain close together, thus forming a perfect snowplow. This technique not only worked, but I now had full control of skiing. This simple little device solved my problem, boosted my confidence, and made skiing fun at last! This anecdote reminds me of how they teach children in Asia to eat with chopsticks—they provide "training chopsticks" that are connected at the top with a cord so kids can learn to keep them together. Also surprisingly helpful for grown Westerners.

Mike, my A-School ski instructor, was thrilled to find out how well I had progressed. Brent, my B-School instructor, told me that he had eaten lunch with Mike the day before, and they had discussed my case and the whole issue of cerebral palsy. Mike had arranged for me to continue in Brent's class but wanted to ensure a "win" for me since I had been so down and frustrated the day before. He knew I was determined to conquer this problem of skiing, and he encouraged me to not give up. Brent came up with the idea of this little device and told Mike that this would solve my problem. What a novel approach!

Sesame Street West was our first run again, to get a feel for the slope and demonstrate how much everybody had remembered. This was the first run with my little device attached to my skis. I not only made it down without any help, but I made it down under full control, with a big smile on my face.

Until then, I had never experienced skiing like that. I did the run again, and I was actually able to relax, look around a bit, and enjoy myself as I looked at the beautiful mountain scenery. I was so happy.

After lunch, we set out for Patrolman #47 and Over Easy #48. These slopes were steeper and higher, and a bit more challenging for me. Afterwards, I could not believe I had done a steep run. From that point on, there would be no more "Sesame Street" runs for me! We practiced our turns, cuts, and stops using both the wedge and the cut technique. I did great on my turn-ins with the help of Mr. Edgie Wedgie, and I hoped this would ultimately help train my right side to ski correctly.

After class, Brent Allen met up with me to see how I was progressing. He told me that he was also adopted. He understood the struggles and challenges I was now facing in life, and he was quite moved by my strong determination to succeed where others might just decide to quit and give up. I was grateful for Brent and Mike for helping this young kid with CP develop self-confidence to snow ski. Looking back on this skiing adventure many years later, I am still amazed at the work and dedication of these two ski instructors—they had encouraged a young skier to look past his perceived limitations. They used innovative techniques to encourage this timid (and often frustrated) beginner to overcome his physical difficulties on the ski slopes. This novel approach planted the mustard seed for what would ultimately develop into my transformation, reaching far beyond that young man on the slopes with his Edgie Wedgie.

On my third day, I was off to C-School! I was stoked! That day's ski lesson was with David, and his class was extremely aggressive and tiring. We first went down Jill's Run #54 and Saint Moritz #46. Then we went down Stumps Alley #45—my first "blue" run! David took off my training aid to see how much control I could execute without it. I was scared, but I did better than I thought. However, it was still not enough to keep control, so he put it back on my skis. I was relieved to have my "friend" back in place to help me down the mountain. Like Linus in the *Peanuts* comics, I still needed my security blanket.

We then went back down Stumps Alley. We worked on turns and more side control and speed. It was fun picking up speed, going faster than I'd ever gone before. My skis started to bounce off the ground as I flew down the mountain, and I felt like I was going a million miles an hour (okay, not literally, but it felt really fast). I was in full control, and it felt great! The weather that afternoon was almost blizzard conditions, and plenty of fresh powder covered the slopes. This was more of a challenge for me since I had never skied in powder before, but I handled it well. By the end of the day, close to three feet of new powder had fallen.

It was awesome up on the slopes that afternoon, not only because of the steep slopes I had conquered but also because the snow and weather conditions were breathtaking. It reminded me of a James Bond movie with James at an exotic mountaintop chateau, ready for some thrilling adventure on the slopes, and of course, I was James Bond in this narrative.

Our class ended midafternoon; however, I went back down Jill's Run #54 and Saint Moritz #46 by myself. I did both of these runs two more times before the lifts closed. It was so cool to finally make a run on my own. For the last runs I took, no one was on the slopes because of the intense, harsh weather. But I did not care; I had triumphed over this mountain, and I wanted to stay here forever.

The fourth day, December 29, the mountain was closed. Blizzard and white-out conditions made it impossible to ski. I was grateful for a day of rest, even if I would not admit it at the time.

The blizzard had subsided the following day. So I spent December 30 skiing with the family. We skied for two hours—just Dad, Chris, and me. This time was special; an activity like this was something I could never do before. I so desperately wanted to show off my new skiing skills. We skied Jill's Run but with a twist at the end. Instead of coming down to the left from the run the normal way, like before, we came down the steep way. We went down Stumps Alley to Chair #2 twice, then down Broadway. The powder was thick and great. I think my dad was even a bit impressed by my skiing. I fell three times due to cutting too sharp, catching powder, and losing my balance on my right side. It was neat to fall in powder; however, getting up was challenging, as I had to position my poles under me and use every ounce of upper-body strength to rise. Fortunately, this was something I had learned well in ski school.

It was a great day to end an uplifting ski trip. I had really exerted myself and was able to show off my new skiing skills to Dad and my stepbrother.

POWDER AND SUCCESS IN UTAH

I would not have another opportunity to snow ski until 1998, at the age of thirty-one. My stepbrother, Chris, was now living in Salt Lake City, Utah. I was still nervous about skiing due to CP. Once again, I enrolled in adult ski school, armed with my Edgie Wedgie. Ski school was a good refresher, but I still wasn't as strong on my right side as I needed to be to form a plow. My instructors gave me some conditioning exercises to do after I left Mammoth

Lakes, which I could do the rest of the year to try to strengthen my leg muscles. But living in Texas, with no real hope of skiing that next winter, I wasn't motivated to do the exercises.

In early 1999, I underwent bunionectomy surgery on my right foot to correct an excruciating bunion on my big toe. Doctors told me that due to CP, an inability to consciously bend my toes, and having flat feet, my right-side toe muscles were way too weak to keep my big toe in proper alignment. Over the years, this had become a painful problem. My bunionectomy and toe realignment surgery fixed everything, even more than I had thought it would. The doctors shaved off my bunion and broke my big toe bones in six places, all the way up to my ankle area, and pinned and screwed them into proper place. It took over eight months for my right foot to fully heal and for my big toe to calm down and lie flat and straight on the floor when I would stand.

That next winter, during snow skiing season with Chris's family, I skied better than I had ever done in my life. And to top it off, I no longer needed Mr. Edgie Wedgie. I was floored! How could realignment of a big toe bring such radical change? This was what I came to call my first "formal experience" of transformation with CP. However, it would take years to fully uncover the reasons for improvement in my skiing ability, ultimately leading me on my current path toward the athlete and bodybuilder I have become today.

Scott Falls
from a Plane

From the depths of the oceans, through the snow-filled mountain slopes, to the skies above, I have always loved three-dimensional activities.

One evening in the dorms at Texas Tech, doing one of my many loads of laundry, I came upon a flyer posted in our laundry room. "Come learn to skydive with Westex Skysports. Holden Hall, November 15–17," it said. I had always had a crazy desire to jump out of an airplane. Skydiving sounded like fun and technically challenging, and I am all about learning and experiencing technically challenging things. But could a kid with CP actually learn to solo skydive? *Could I, would I, will I skydive?*

Over the next week, I thought about skydiving, daydreamed about skydiving, and even went to the library to research skydiving. After all, these were the pre-Google, pre-internet days, when you couldn't search online from the confines of your dorm room as we can today. I even talked about skydiving to several close friends in my dorm. Most of them said that I would not be allowed to jump, that I would not be *able* to jump, or that I would back down before my first jump. I tried to talk some of my friends into taking the class with me, but they all said no, and they assumed I would let it go. This kind of talk not only infuriated me but also made me even more determined to learn to skydive.

I called home and, as gingerly as a nervous son could, informed Mom that I was going to sign up for lessons. At first Mom said absolutely not, under no circumstances was I going to do a silly thing like that! But over time, and several follow-up phone calls, Mom came to know that I was determined to do it and that I was preparing as only a well-trained engineering student would: safety first.

That very next day, I saw a friend with whom I had served in the residence halls association as a senator the year before. Toby and I talked about skydiving, and he confided in me some very encouraging news. Not only did he say that I would have no problem at all with my CP but also that he had taken this very same training from the people at Westex Skysports. These guys were pros and knew what they were doing, he told me. He'd had a blast. He even said that if I brought a VCR tape with me, they would record my jump. This sealed the deal. Scotty, CP or not, was going to learn to skydive! Toby's positive feedback and encouragement was what this shy guy with CP needed to press forward.

On November 15, 1990, skydiving class started. I felt butterflies in my stomach as I walked the three long blocks from my dorm to Holden Hall. Every step felt like gravity was increasing and my feet were getting harder and harder to lift. However, my upper body was in an all-out fight with my lower body to get to this class with haste.

Upon arriving, I saw that the class was full of wide-eyed kids just like me, nervous and intrigued, looking at all the wonders and sights to be seen. That evening was primarily a demo and introduction session. We first watched a video on skydiving and all kinds of different free falls and formations. They showed us what the class involved and introduced us to all of our would-be skydiving instructors *if* we decided to stick around for the class. This was followed by talks with the instructors, who showed us the parachute rigs we would be using.

Then we saw a video of a lawyer in a suit at a desk, going through all the legalese, and at a predetermined point, he asked us to sign our class registration forms—if we still planned to go through with it. I signed without hesitation. I knew turning in this form would take still more courage. Then the camera panned back as the lawyer stood up from his desk and, along with the cameraman, dropped out of the office door, which was really an airplane door.

We all gasped when he made his grand exit. I was impressed! We received our packets then, which included everything from a bumper sticker to a dive logbook.

The class started the next night, and the plan was that on Saturday, we would go to Stanton, Texas, to the dive zone, or "DZ" as skydivers call it, and dive later that afternoon. We would receive additional instructions on emergency maneuvers and landing techniques. *Sounds like a blast*, I thought. I talked to both Brent Berry and John Pribyla, our skydiving instructors, about my cerebral palsy, and Brent (head instructor) said that it shouldn't pose a problem. He said since I climb and rappel and was an avid scuba diver, he thought I would be just fine. I hoped so. I was a little nervous, but I was really looking forward to this. I paid for the class, turned in my forms, and could not wait for the next day.

November 16—once again, I made my way from Bledsoe, the three blocks to Holden Hall, for skydiving class. That night's walk was somehow easier than the night before. In fact, I may have even run a bit, just to get the best seat in the room. We covered a lot of information that night, such as how the parachutes work and how the harness is attached to the diver, and we got instructions on procedures and processes. We saw more videos on "this and that," like what to do when *this* happens and what to do when *that* happens. I took copious notes. After all, I was learning about how to save my own life in the event of "this or that." By the end of the first evening, we had covered quite a lot of material, but we still had a bit more to cover the following night. The only part that looked really challenging for me was climbing out of the airplane and onto the wheel while holding on to the strut. By the time the night's class was over, many things were flying through my brain at terminal velocity. Most of them were the "ifs." I must admit that I was a bit scared. After all, what sane person would voluntarily jump out of a perfectly good airplane at around four thousand feet? It just wasn't an everyday experience I had under my belt...yet.

November 17—the day started at 6:00 a.m., when we met some fellow students at a restaurant across town and carpooled out to Stanton, Texas, to the Westex Skysports DZ. I had a severe case of butterflies in my stomach, so I only ordered soup for breakfast. We then drove the hundred miles to the DZ, listening to Tom Petty's song "Free Falling." We arrived at about 10:30 a.m. to a small private airport near Stanton.

Our class started as soon as all twelve of us green, newbie skydiver cadets arrived. We began by watching the jumpmaster rig our parachutes and place them into their containers. They had the process down to a simple, systematic, and clean workflow. I was impressed with how simple yet complex this life-saving system really was. We finished the rest of our videotaped lessons and practiced various exit maneuvers along with simulator work, which included "what to do if..." and "when malfunctions occur, you do..."

Their simulator was really the neat part. They would attach you to a jump harness system, hoist you fifteen feet in the air, and then simulate various recovery maneuvers while shaking and rolling the rig with you in it. You can't pay enough for this at an amusement park!

Finally, it was time for the big jump.

There were eight of us jumping from my class. The other four could not or would not jump due to either not passing elements earlier in the day or for other reasons. I would be the first one out the door in the third planeload of skydivers, with three divers per trip. I got suited up with help from our jumpmaster.

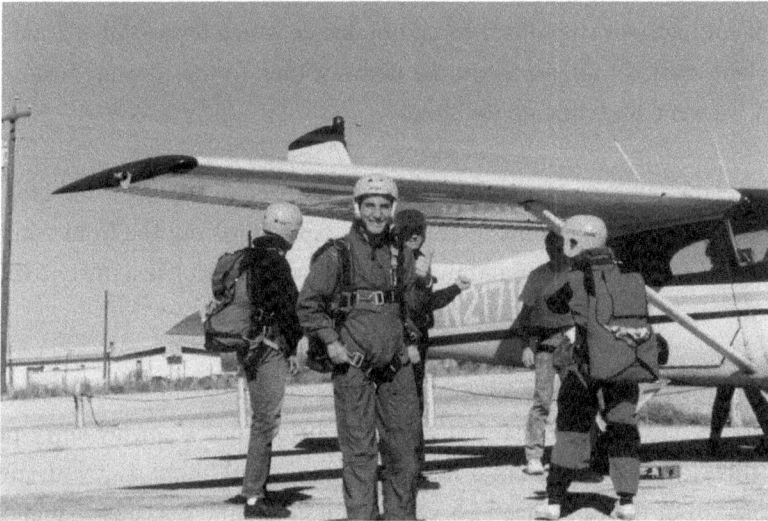

Suited up for my solo skydiving jump

I was fitted in my very own jumpsuit, parachute, and nerdy-looking yellow helmet and goggles. I thought I looked good in my jumpsuit and parachute rigging. The helmet was another story! I often wondered why our jumpmasters did not have to use one of those little yellow acorn-looking things on their heads, yet we did. Also, it was ridiculously hard to walk upright due to the cinched tight-fitting harness straps down below. And the weight of this rig felt like we had bricks on our backs. But that was not going to deter this cadet from climbing aboard. Luckily, they helped us into the plane. I figured the instructors knew by experience that we would all need help embarking.

We loaded the plane in reverse order of our upcoming spectacular exit. I was last to enter the plane. No longer nervous, I was pumped and ready. When the plane took off, I could not see out the front window because I was too far down on the floor (the copilot seat had been removed to make room for skydiving cargo). When the door closed, I heard the pilot yell, "Contact!" over the radio, and suddenly, our little Cessna 182 roared to life as the propeller started to spin. Faster and faster, louder and louder both the plane engine and my heartbeat became. This was the moment! This was the beginning of my test of courage—or stupidity. I could not decide which it was. All of a sudden, the plane started to move down the taxiway, then to the runway. Faster and faster we went, and then up we lifted.

As the plane's altitude increased, the g-force pressed us all down, and I felt my whole body compress to the floor. I so wanted to look out the front window, but since I was on the floor and the plane was at what felt like a thirty-five-de-gree upward angle, this was not possible.

Up, up, up we went. Then we banked right; the change in force pressed me against the closed door that just moments before had been my entry point into this ride. For a moment, I hoped the door would hold shut with me up against it. But then I realized I had a parachute on and nervously laughed at myself for thinking such a thing. This was the only way to fly.

When the plane reached altitude, our pilot gave our divemaster, Brent Barry, the thumbs up. He opened the door. At this point, my heart started beating faster. If it was possible to be any more nervous, I was headed for that moment when I started hearing the wind howl right by my ear. But I knew I was safe. After all, I did have a parachute on, and my jumpmaster was right next to me. So what was there to be nervous about?

I looked out the door. When you are told, "Don't look down," what do you do? *The ground looks mighty small from around 4,200 feet*, I thought as I looked out the open door. For some reason, this didn't concern me as much as I thought it should. In the past, I had often said to others that if I ever went skydiving, you would have trouble getting me out of the plane. But as it turned out, I had trouble staying *in* this plane. I wanted out. I wanted to do this more than ever. It was showtime! I was focused on the task I had been trained so well to perform: getting out of this darn plane.

Slowly and methodically, I scooted my butt over to the door and swung my right foot out. But the wind grabbed my leg and forced it back beyond the door. It took me a moment or two to stabilize my right leg and place my foot onto the wheel platform. I then swung my left foot over and out the door with a little less trouble than my right. I positioned it on the wheel platform next to my right foot. I then reached up with my right hand and grabbed on to the wing strut as hard as I could while holding on to the doorframe with my stronger left hand.

Inching my butt closer to the door, I moved my left hand out into the wind, still holding on to the strut as hard as I could. I then stood up on the wheel well platform and inched my butt all the way out the door. The wind was rushing past my head, making lots of noise. Looking straight ahead, I saw the propeller going around and around, really fast. I heard the wind and our buzzing engine keeping us up in the sky with fierce force. With my right hand, I was to reach as far up the strut as I could while taking my right foot off the wheel well and then do the same with my left hand. At this point I would be "flying" like Superman, holding on to the plane by the right-side strut.

As reality soon came crashing back into focus, however, this was not the way it happened upon my exit. I did manage to get out of the plane and onto the wheel platform while holding on to the strut. But when my right hand tried to reach farther up the strut, I could no longer keep its weak grip, and it slipped loose off the strut. I found myself dangling by my left hand like a monkey at the zoo. I took a quick look down at the small plots of land way beyond my feet, then I looked up to figure out why I had let go of the strut with my right hand. Okay, I thought, I could just reach up and grab the strut with my right hand, and all would be fine once again. However, upon doing so, my body turned farther to the right due to the wind. This resulted in my right hand moving farther from the strut as I turned, with my back now against the open door.

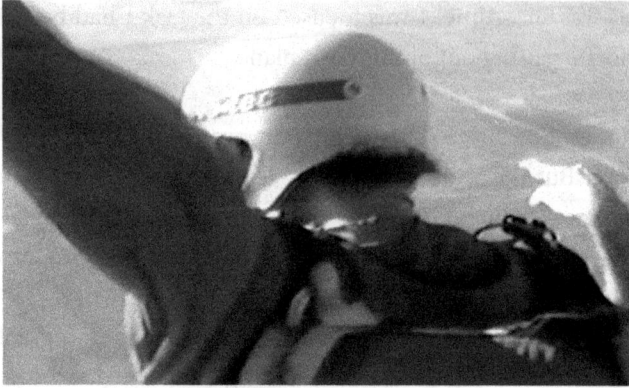

Trying to hold on to the strut of a Cessna 182 while skydiving

My mind conjured up memories of the playground at Eanes during PE, where the coaches would drill me, and the other kids would laugh at me hanging on that chin-up bar by my left, *strong arm* only—apparently, *Monkey Boy* was now about to skydive.

Yet, at close to 4,200 feet off the ground, this thought made me smile. *I'm actually about to skydive*, I thought. *How many of those kids could, or rather would, do that today?* Meanwhile, back in reality, during all this internal memory-lane strategizing and maneuvering, my jumpmaster was yelling at the top of his lungs, "Jump, jump, jump!" I could not see or hear him due to the circus act I was performing in front of him. All I heard was wind noise and the pounding of my heart.

I soon realized that reaching my right hand up to the strut was not going to work, so I decided the best I could do was start my jump follow-through to the best of my ability while in this odd position. I let go with my left hand and formed the classic skydiver's "hard X pattern" that the instructors had taught us in class. As I released my grip, I saw the Cessna 182 that I was just holding on to begin to get small, as if it was moving up and away from me very fast. I started counting: "Arch one thousand…two one thousand…three one thousand…four one thousand…five one thousand…throw one thousand."

I looked up, and there popped out my main chute. As I saw my slider sliding down into place above my head, I thanked God that everything was in its proper place. My ram-air class Manta 288 canopy was such a beautiful sight. I thanked God again for this perfect, beautiful canopy, which was properly inflated and ready to be released from one-quarter break position. I yelled a loud "Woo hoo!" as those on the ground later told me.

All right! Everything is cool! Back to the plan.

I found the toggles with both hands at exactly the same time, released the brakes, flared my chute, and found the arrow I was supposed to follow all the way to the ground. I could not see it at first by looking over my shoulders or underneath me, so I maneuvered a one-half break left. There I found it, and following its instruction, I aligned myself to its direction.

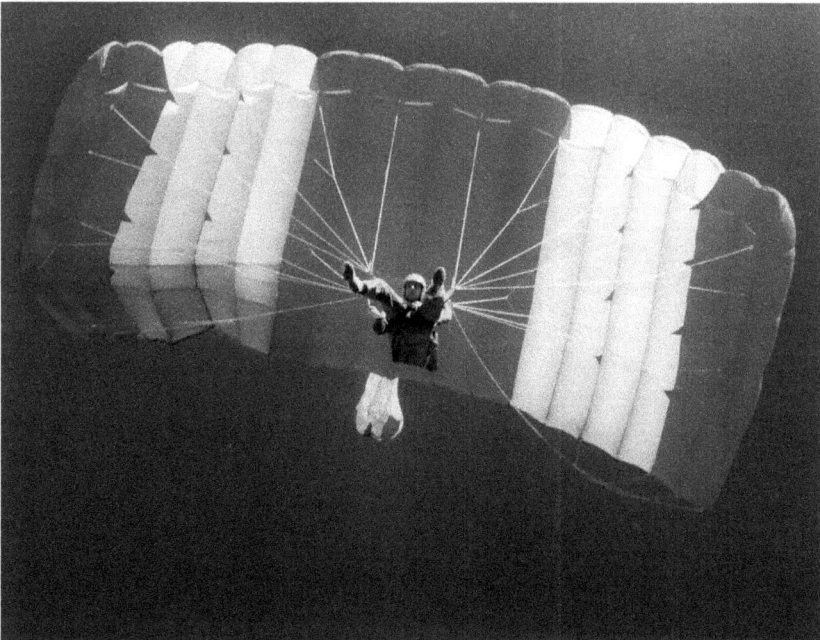

Coming in for a landing after first jump

It struck me as funny to see my tennis shoes and legs dangling 3,200 feet off the ground. This was not a usual sight for me but very thrilling nonetheless. I followed my training and kept my parachute in alignment with the big white arrow that kept me on course far below. I descended and even made a running-style touchdown landing, running a bit before I released one toggle to collapse my shoot. The goal was to land within fifty feet of the arrow. I accomplished a perfect landing, right on target—just ten feet away! I was not only in the landing zone but also right on the bull's-eye with my first jump.

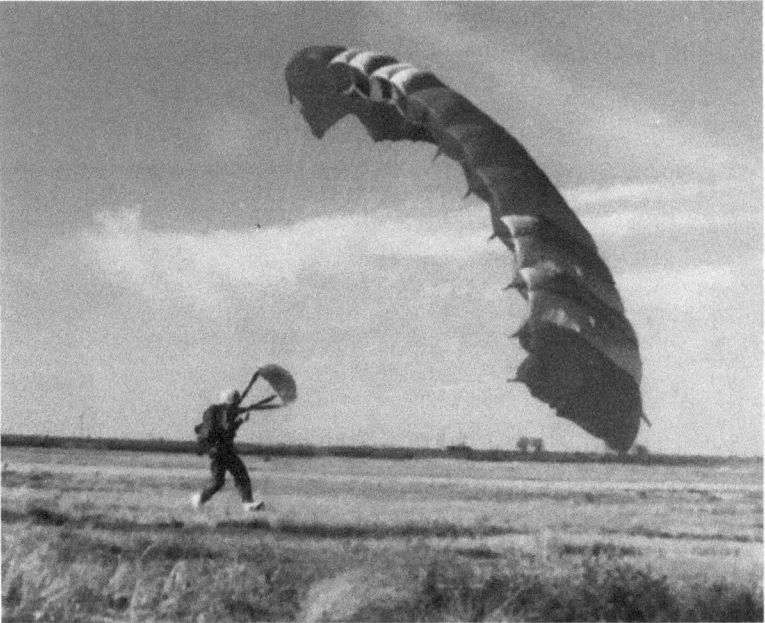

Making a running landing on first jump

When I landed, a friend took a photograph of me holding my parachute wadded up in my arms.

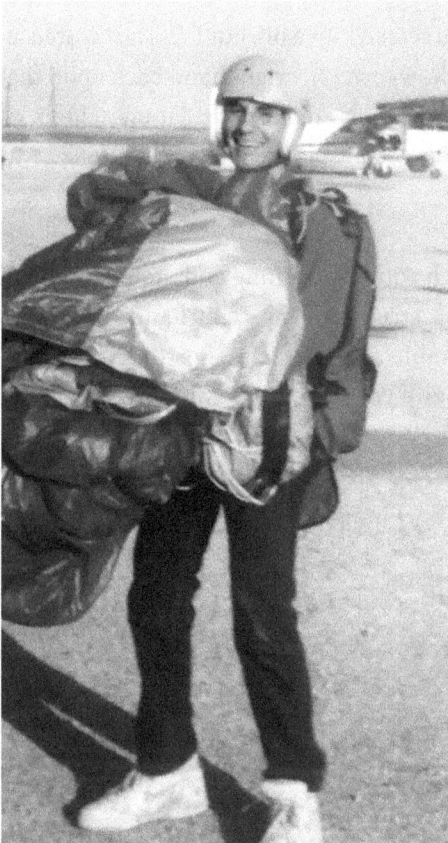

Solo skydiving jump landing

I had the biggest grin on my face. I had made my very first accelerated free fall and solo skydiving jump. CP did not stop this guy. What a rush! I could not wait to go back up and do it again, to glide through the air again, free like a bird.

During my debrief, Brent, my jumpmaster, said I needed to work on keeping hold of the strut so I could achieve a better "arch" position. But he thought I had particularly good canopy control and a great exit, despite his ordering me to jump when my right hand lost grip, and good pull maneuvering.

I think I might have scared him a bit, but I was not scared at all, hanging in the air, contemplating how to get my right hand back up to that strut. He proudly signed my logbook with an added note: "Tough climb out but you tried to get front. Good canopy control. Brent Berry DW-688." I was stoked. My first jump signed off.

I'd followed through with my training and did not panic when I prematurely let go of that plane strut with my right hand. I'd made the best of it and did not spin or tumble at all, which tends to lead to entanglement of your canopy strings around your legs, something we'd practiced on the simulator all morning long.

I was eager for my next jump.

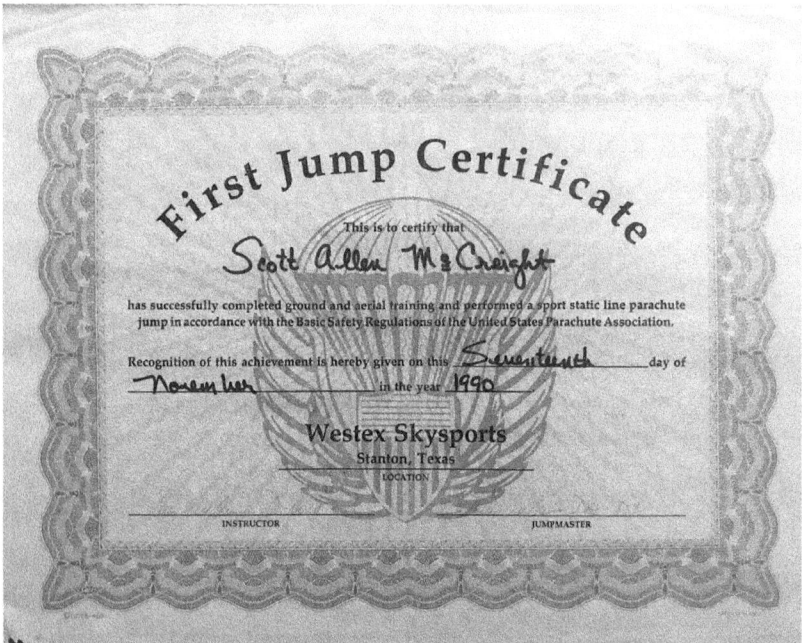

First solo jump certificate

That night, I called Mom and Dad to tell them the news, that I had become a skydiver. During the call, I held on to my signed copy of my solo jump certificate, a certificate I have framed and mounted on the wall right below a picture of my first jump, canopy in midair, still on display today.

Brent had been correct. He had said that right after you make your first jump, you are hooked. You are going to want to jump again and again, finding yourself thinking about skydiving in class and figuring out wind speed, wind direction, and when is the best time to dive again.

Over the next couple of weeks, it indeed seemed like that was *all* I wanted to do. Many of my friends in the dorm were asking questions about my jump. Even Doug, my hall director, wanted information on skydiving. Dad took the news pretty well. He said he wanted to see my logbook and all the material when I came to visit at Christmas. Deep down inside, I think he was proud that his son with CP had become a skydiver.

I continued to skydive for the next year of school when I had time and money to jump. Over time, my exits did improve, and with a modified foot "tip-off" maneuver, I was successful at deploying with only a little trouble with upper-body strength and coordination. But I never quite mastered the process, and once again this dream was put on hold, shelved, and almost forgotten, for I would not get another opportunity to return to skydiving until 2019, thirty years later.[31]

THE SHIFT TO INDUSTRIAL SYSTEMS ENGINEERING

During the summer of my (first) junior year of college, I took a job as an engineer with the Department of Defense (DoD) in Southern California. I not only worked in the field that I was studying but also had a passion for the technology I was designing and building. I worked with some very sophisticated and highly classified communication systems and technology that seemed right up my alley as an electrical engineering student. I even designed, built out, and procured the MARS and CAP radio systems for three bases under our command. I designed the commands' Telecommunication Disaster Preparedness and Control Plan and even worked with fiber communication systems and telephony equipment that was quite state of the art. Putting my love of radio and electronics to work in such an interesting field was in itself very exciting.

During this first stint at the DoD, Don Owen, the head of our division (Code 053) took a special interest in my abilities and drive. He also happened to be an engineering graduate of Texas Tech. He was an industrial engineer (IE) and led the team of IEs to which I was assigned. Over the next three summers, I was assigned more and more IE-related projects that dealt with human factors and ergonomics, to name just a few. I was intrigued that an engineer could possess "people skills" as well as technological knowledge all in a single degree. In the early days of my DoD career, I primarily only worked with technology by myself. However, as an IE, I was on a team with other IEs, and I learned that I liked working with people and technology together. I wanted to return to Texas Tech and look into the industrial engineering program. How could I combine IE and EE into a career like this? As it turned out, my division head had done his job, his recruitment of me as another IE into his ranks.

GRADUATION DAY

Graduation from college was finally at hand. After five years of the most life-changing and growth-extending experiences I'd fought hard to obtain, the day had finally arrived. Back in high school, "they" had said this day would never happen. They said a guy with CP would not be able to go to college, much less graduate with a degree—an engineering degree at that. I was extremely proud to prove all those people wrong as I walked across that stage at Texas Tech University and received my diploma for a bachelor of science in industrial engineering.

Both my mom and dad and the rest of my family were proud too. I had come so far from the days of shyness, introversion, and self-doubt about what I could achieve. There I was, walking across that stage when my name was called. Something that I thought, as a high school kid with CP, I would never get to do. My only concerns at that moment were making sure not to trip on my oversized gown and carrying out a firm handshake with my right hand.

PART 3

Finding Faith

Even Mustard-Seed-Sized Faith
Can Move Mountains

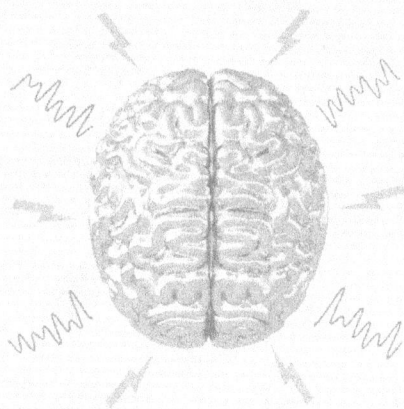

I Can Do All Things

FAITH AND HOPE HAVE PLAYED A MAJOR ROLE IN MY TRANSFORMATION, both spiritually and emotionally. It was the new millennium, spring of 2000. I was enjoying the great outdoors on a daylong hike with my good friend Lonnie Wendling, out at Enchanted Rock in the Texas Hill Country. Lonnie had recently relocated from Texas to Northern California with a high-tech company that we had both worked for in the not-so-distant past. He had taken a job out West while I stayed in Austin, and he had come back for a long weekend to hike with me.

We had hung out together over many years in the past, in Northern California as well as Austin—spending a lot of time outdoors on scuba diving adventures and on hikes like the one we were partaking in that day. My physical transformation had not yet started, so hiking was more difficult for me than for Lonnie. However, this had never stopped me from getting outdoors and spending time on the trail with a good friend. We spent time catching up on what life was now like for each of us. Far from the days of drinking, hot tub parties, and weekend "diversions" of our youth, this hike turned out to be the beginning of my spiritual transformation. At that time, I had begun to question the meaning of life but had not yet shared this introspection with any of my friends, including Lonnie. A few miles into our hike, Lonnie and I stopped at a rock outcropping to rest and have a bite to eat. Lonnie reached into his backpack and handed me a book and told me that I would enjoy reading it. A bit taken aback, I reluctantly agreed to read his book. I was surprised at the fact that not only had he packed such a book on this particular hike but that he suggested I read it. After all, up to this point, our friendship had never included reading books. This book, written by Tim LaHaye and Jerry B. Jenkins, was titled *Left Behind*. Lonnie said little, other than to read the book and pass it along.

Over the next month, I read not only *Left Behind* but also *This Present Darkness* by Frank E. Peretti, a book that another good friend had gifted to me. Up to this point in my life, I was not an avid reader, so these reading requests seemed a bit odd. However, I was beginning to see patterns developing all around me in all different aspects of my life. Chance or happenstance had never seemed this strong a "coincidence" before—but it was too strong to be just that. I wanted to know more, to understand more, to be more than what I currently was.

Coming to faith in Christ occurred shortly after, at age thirty-three. The irony of this number is not lost on me. Thirty-three was the age Jesus was when he died on the cross. The year was 2001, September 5, to be exact. I remember this day well because just six days later, on September 11, the twin towers fell in New York, which forever changed the lives of everyone. September 5 had not been a notable day for me, other than the willful act of giving up the silly idea that I had to *do* something or *be* something I was not, in order to make it in life or fit into a specific group or demographic of people. I had been so determined to be a "normal person" and to fit in, but it was just not working. I could not "fix" my CP or ignore my condition to be what I thought I needed to be. I could no longer carry the weight of what I thought I "should" do, bootstrapping my way through life.

It is quite an eye-opener once you're on the other side of faith, as you can see things in a whole new light. I guess that's why I have heard the saying "looking through a glass darkly" when referring to something unseen for what it's really worth, usually through the eyes of someone who has the incorrect or incomplete picture at the time. I now understand that God had prepared me for just *this* moment, and it was time to bring me in to understanding His plan, His fold…for He had gotten my attention by allowing me to be in positions that I could no longer bootstrap it through. I thought about the expression "pride goeth before the fall." Trying to do it my way, I was tired. It was exhausting all the time. It was time to do a complete overhaul on who I really needed to be and what I would do next. Reading the books *Left Behind* and *This Present Darkness*, along with many others, and experiencing many inexplicable encounters in my life allowed me to reimagine what I was actually a part of— something much bigger than I could ever fully know.

ON THE TRAIL

During the weeks leading up to and including March 7 through March 15, 2002, my faith was boosted to a new level, strengthened, and expanded as a result of a special nine-day hiking and camping trip into the Grand Canyon with a group of singles—young adults from my new church. I was one of the most unlikely candidates to ever be part of a group of avid, experienced hikers on an adventure like this. One that I had long thought I could never accomplish—at least, not on this *grand* scale. I knew I was unlikely to be chosen for the trip because of my CP limitations as well as my lack of hiking experience and, quite honestly, the lack of length and depth of my budding Christian faith. Due to my fondness for the outdoors and hiking, I really wanted to go, and I had learned that God does not choose the equipped but equips His chosen. God had showed me that we can dream big. I just never expected my dream to be as big as the Grand Canyon!

The Grand Canyon is one of the seven natural wonders of the world and one of our planet's most astounding features. The sheer majesty and beauty of the scenery is beyond belief. I was awed by all the details I learned.

The skill rating for this trip was "expert hiking and primitive camping." In other words, for serious hikers only. I trained with a team for months for this trip. I learned extremely fast that you cannot accomplish a trek like this without proper training, preparation, and most of all, a serious concern for safety.

IN THE CANYON

This Grand Canyon adventure was sponsored by First Evangelical Free Church (now known as Austin Oaks Church), as part of their Impact Singles Spring Break, and I felt strongly led to be a part of this adventure. The group consisted of more than forty people divided into seven smaller hiking teams called cells. Traveling from Austin to this faraway land took us nearly twenty hours by charter bus, beginning in the very early hours of the morning. Norton, our staff leader, had been a major sponsor of this trip and had taken guided tours like this one for many years. He had the right connections for obtaining the proper permits and paying the correct fees that would allow us to explore down into this deep, vast canyon.

All seven hiking teams, a.k.a. cells, were given different trails to hike and explore over a six-day period. Each cell consisted of six to twelve people with a varying range of skill and endurance levels. The team I was paired up with consisted of six people and received one of the most challenging and difficult routes to follow. My team hiked and trained together for over four months in and around our local area of Austin prior to this adventure. We learned proper techniques for hiking the Canyon and proper backpack selection and weighting. And we participated in team-building exercises and other wilderness survival skills, including dress and emergency procedures. Mike and Keith were our leaders and were very experienced and knowledgeable about this type of adventure; our team could not have done this trip without their help, support, and expert guidance. This became apparent from the moment we descended into the canyon.

On the South Rim, the weather was below freezing, with patches of snow. In the canyon, however, it was dry and sunny, in the upper sixties in the daytime and lows in the forties at night—ideal for camping.

Arrival at the Canyon

Arriving at the Canyon the night before, we made our final preparations for descending early the next morning along with one final "real" meal, shower, and rest. Our team leaders went over last-minute safety facts, rules, and instructions as well as gear and backpack inspections. They went through each of our backpacks and weighed everything on a hanging scale. I thought it was so strange that they would weigh everything. But it was something I would later praise God for, as my pack would have been way too heavy for me. Many of my items were loaded back on the bus. Due to the imbalance between my stronger left side and weaker, spastic right side, my pack was fitted for fifty pounds. Others' were heavier, while some of our smaller-framed members had lighter packs than mine. Due to the anticipated stresses my body would likely encounter as we hiked farther into the canyon, my leaders wanted to make sure I had supplies in my pack that would become lighter as our trip progressed, so I carried most of the food for our team.

Day 1: The Descent

Early the next morning, my team descended into the Grand Canyon at Hermits Rest at 6,700 feet. We followed Hermit Trail to Santa Maria Spring, where we stopped and pulled water from the springs and took a small snack break. We readjusted packs and straps and checked for hot spots on our feet. We stopped for lunch at Lookout Point, then continued the trail past Breezy Point and descended the Cathedral Stairs around Cope Butte to the Tonto Trail at 3,200 feet.

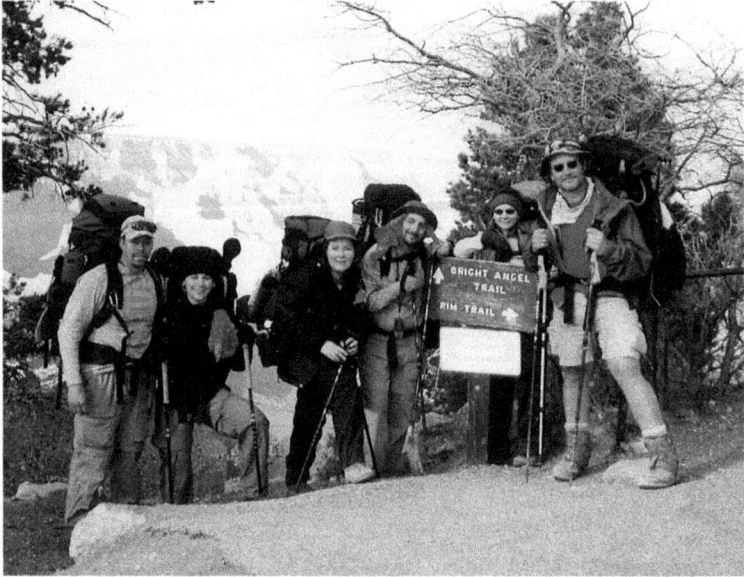

With the Grand Canyon hiking team
(Left to right: Mike, Jodie, Darla, me, Liz, and Keith)

After constant downhill hiking with a full pack and poles, I was really starting to feel my legs burn. I was using my poles not only to keep me upright and stable but also as crutches to just walk. I had serious pain and muscle cramps by this point. It felt like I had polio and I was losing my ability to walk. Mike encouraged me by telling me that I was doing great, that there were only a couple of miles left until we reached camp at Monument Creek. At one point, Mike would run ahead with his full pack, drop the pack, and run back to where I was, traveling at a snail's pace. He'd take my backpack, then walk with me to his pack, all the while encouraging me, repeating this until we reached our campsite two miles away. What a burden he took upon himself for me. I was relying on faith and Mike's help to make it to camp and praying that my body, my legs in particular, would hold up and deliver me to camp. I would later refer to this as my "coming to Jesus" moment, relying totally on Him for providing strength and deliverance. Faith always pays dividends!

By the time Mike and I made it to camp (#1 on the West Region map), the team had set up camp, and all were cheering me on for making it. To this day, Mike will always have a special place in my heart for lightening my load as well as keeping my spirits high. Mike, Keith, and I discussed my pain; they prayed over me and told me that the next day would be a new and exceptionally light day. Only about a mile down Monument Creek to the Colorado River at 2,369 feet. I was extremely grateful for such a short remaining distance to hike because my legs were all but seized up by this time. How would I make it one more step? I needed time to recover. I needed a miracle.

Day 2: The Final Descent to the Bottom

I awoke early in extreme pain, but it was still not as bad as the day before had been. I was grateful to be alive. I downed another dose of Celebrex that my primary care doctor had the foresight to prescribe and I had the foresight to pack for the trip. I began the task of learning how to walk all over again, albeit it only over to the breakfast area at camp. It felt like ten thousand miles, with legs made of unset Jell-O and pins and needles piercing every nerve fiber in my body. My CP was really acting spastic too.

As we hoisted the packs once again and began the trek, I was placed in front of the team, and our pace was slow and steady down the jagged Monument Creek Trail. Everyone was taking in the splendor of the canyon view. Everyone, that is, except me. I was intensely concentrating on the scene from that stop-motion animated Christmas film *Santa Claus Is Comin' to Town* by Jules Bass and Arthur Rankin Jr. All I could do was keep reciting to myself, *Put one foot in front of the other*, as I slowly and painfully moved down the trail. And I prayed. Two hours later, we reached camp (#2 on the West Region map). I was so grateful for making it to the valley floor. I had made it to the bottom of the Grand Canyon…alive!

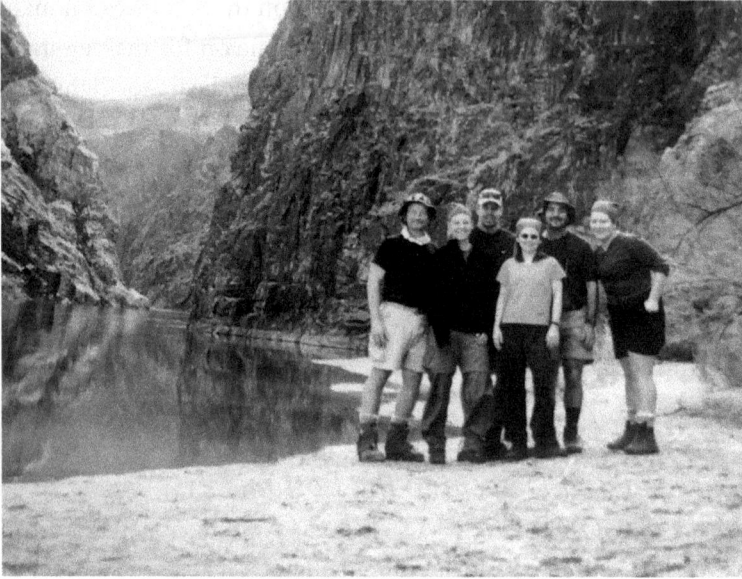

At the bottom of the Grand Canyon
(Left to right: Keith, Jodie, Mike, Liz, me, and Darla)

Day 3: The Climb Begins

On the third day, I was feeling much better. Still sore, but my muscles were beginning to respond to my brain in a more organized and predictable manner. Breakfast was more refreshing than the past two mornings. This was partly due to hunger and needing protein for repairing my body and partly due to feeling alive, really alive, for the first time. After all, I was in a place that few would ever be able to go, with a group of people who were supporting each other both physically and spiritually. I couldn't help but feel extremely grateful for this life I had been granted.

We even found an outhouse with a real toilet seat. No walls, but an actual latrine. After three days of digging and bagging up everything (pack out what you pack in), this was a welcome stop. And what a view! Sitting there on the throne overlooking the Salt Creek and the canyon far below, with the canyon wall and rim behind me, it was so peaceful and relaxing. Or at least for a while, until I'd hear a faint bus, a loud car, or a dog barking some 3,600 feet up the cliff behind me on the South Rim at Mohave Point Overlook. I can only imagine gazing through high-powered binoculars or camera lenses and spotting a hiker sitting all alone, doing his business far below. What a moment killer for me! But I had to laugh. After all, it *was* hilarious. I continued my restful sit, taking in the vista.

After breakfast, our group broke camp and trekked back to where we'd spent the first night, then over to Cedar Springs and out to a fantastic overlook for lunch, where we took in a splendid view of the valley floor. I thought about how, *just that morning* (off to our left), we were 1,031 feet below. After lunch, we mounted packs and headed around the east side of the Inferno to Salt Creek (#3), right off the Tonto Trail, where we camped that night. Upon arriving, we were told that we could not pull water from this creek due to low levels of uranium in the water. I had not known there was radioactive uranium in the Grand Canyon. I hoped we didn't glow after that night.

Day 4: Cold Returns as We Ascend

On the way back up the Tonto Trail at 3,560 feet, we hit a thunderstorm and a cold front that pushed temperatures down fifteen degrees. We ate lunch at Dana Butte, looking over at the Colorado River far below. This part of the trail was flat and sparse. I was hiking behind Liz, the smallest and lightest member of our team, when a big wind gust swooped down, picked her up, and moved her quite a distance down the Tonto Trail. Her feet once again returned to the earth as easily as an astronaut would bounce down a trail on the moon. Later that evening on our debrief of the day, she said she had been struggling with the weight and asked God to lighten her load and "move her lightly down the trail." If I had not been right behind her, witnessing it with my own eyes, I don't know if I could fathom this event. We hiked over to Horn Creek (#4 on my East Region map) and spent the night underneath a fast-moving thunderstorm. The night was incredibly windy and rainy. Toward the higher elevations on the Bright Angel Trail, we had to don our winter coats and secure our crampons (ice cleats) due to the snow and ice.

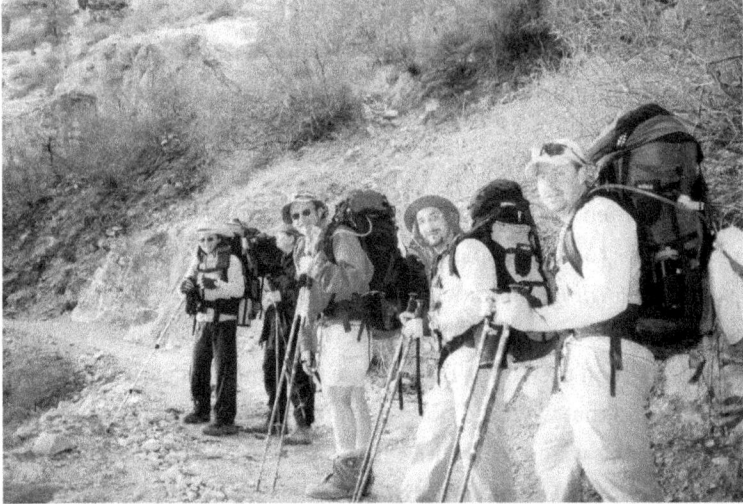

On the trail of the Grand Canyon
(Left to right: Liz, Jodie, Keith, me, and Mike)

Day 5: The Climb

We broke camp early and hiked to a very windy Plato Point at the far end of the Bright Angel Trail, then all the way up the Bright Angel Trail past Indian Garden, where we took our lunch. Then we went up the steep, winding trail next to Garden Creek to the club house and up, up to the visitor center on the South Rim of the canyon. This part of the trek was crowded with travelers and tourists. Lots of ice and snow covered the trail, so we kept our crampons on for traction and stability. Some tourists were on mules, and I could not help but think who was safer: us with boots and crampons or those travelers on mules? One wrong move and it was off the side, a long drop. With all the mule urine and ice on the trail, I was glad for my crampons and sturdy hiking boots. It was slow going, but we made it.

At the rim, we caught a bus from the visitor center over to our "base camp." I can only surmise that after six days in the Grand Canyon with no showers, sweating and all, we must have smelled pretty ripe to the others on that bus. I was even offended by my own aroma. But we all made it, rim to water to rim! This guy with CP experienced hiking the Grand Canyon, both body and faith strengthened by what only Christ can do. That final night we spent back at "base camp" after a long shower and a good home-cooked meal topside, grateful for civilization, provisions, and hot water.

We had hiked 26.8 horizontal miles and over 9,000 vertical feet in six days. This was an adventure that would be difficult for anyone, even more so for a young man with CP. God had once again carried me through an adventure and refined and deepened my faith.

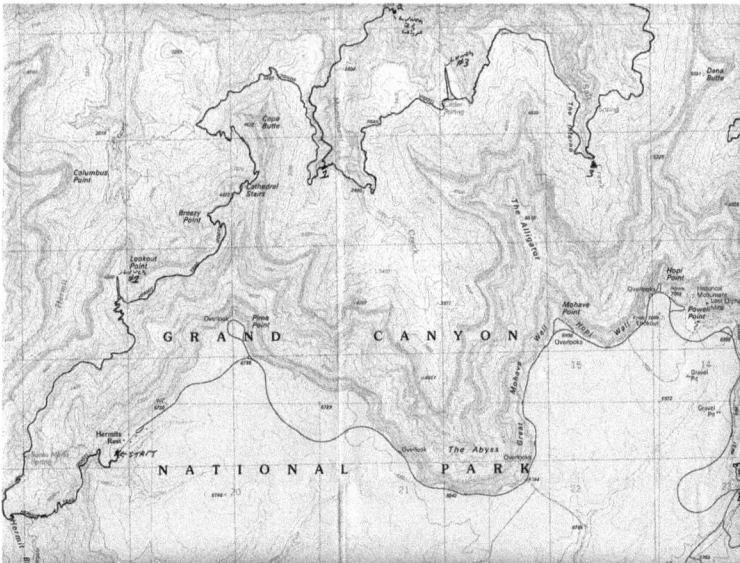

Grand Canyon hiking map of where we hiked: where we started
(from the west moving east)

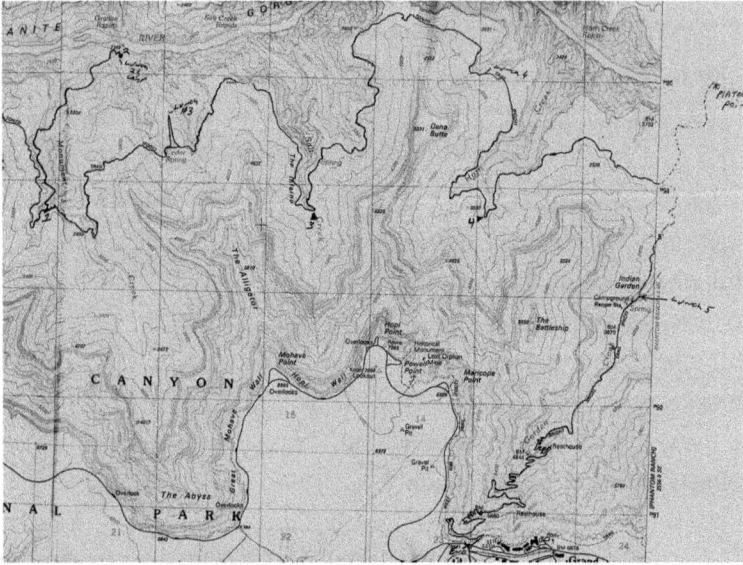

Grand Canyon hiking map: where we went
(ending up at the east end of this trail)

PART 4

The Suffering and Breakthroughs

*Discovering a New Way
to Live Life to the Fullest*

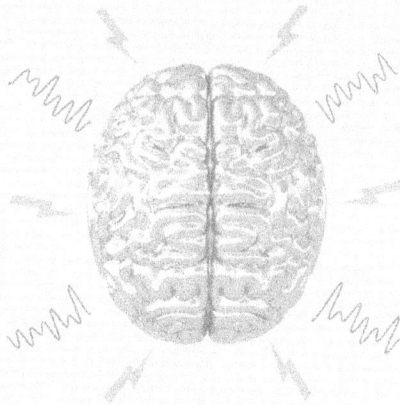

Complacency Can Kill

IN 1999, ABOUT SIX YEARS AFTER MY UNDERGRADUATE SCHOOL ENDED and the formal "learning" had slowed down, a very sinister thought began to nest in my brain. Or perhaps it grew from a seed that had been planted there long, long ago. Maybe the seed was there all along, from my early childhood. This sinister seed went by the name of complacency. Subtle in nature, persistent, and always there nudging me, as a deceptive, persuasive voice would, laying down little evil thoughts. Thoughts such as "I can't, so why try?"

This complacency was so dark and so hideous that it not only snuck up on me but almost completely devoured me before I even knew it. After all my triumphs and challenges undertaken and won, and adventures that most people, let alone folks with cerebral palsy, would likely never dare to undertake, I started subconsciously believing this sinister foe called complacency—that force that feeds us the lie "I can't, so why try?"

I soon found myself in the doldrums of life, post-school, working long hours for high-tech companies. As a senior engineer and technologist, I designed and built multimillion-dollar semiconductor manufacturing systems, engineered innovative ways not only to design but also to manufacture very complex semiconductor equipment, and managed multiple $100 million products as an engineering program manager. It all seemed exciting and fulfilling on the

141

surface, but deep down inside, it held little long-term motivation for me in "my mission" in life. I was successful at my various positions and performed at a very high level. However, I lacked motivation or drive outside of work. For a while, all I had was my work life. Success at work does not necessarily translate to success outside work—and then came a lack of exercise and long travel and work schedules to bog down the soul, and complacency took root.

When you stop learning, you stop living, and when you stop living, that's when complacency really sneaks up on you for the kill. This was something I had come to understand throughout all the past adventures, challenges, and triumphs in my life. Some of these adventures even trained this message into me literally, because if you become complacent in a sport, like cave scuba diving or skydiving, for example, you will die! This philosophy was ingrained in everything I did, and most of my friends heard it echoed whenever they were around me. However, in the years that would follow, complacency grew in my everyday life by small amounts until it nearly took me out altogether.

I would soon learn how sinister and subtle complacency could be. To overcome it, I would have to learn to start believing in myself all over again. I would have to simply put my brain in my locker (more on this later) and just listen and do what needed to be done to create a new, improved version of me.

I CAN'T, SO WHY TRY?

Faith and hope are strong friends to have around. However, when you misplace these two powerful friends, anxiety and depression show up every time. In my case, I think God was using these uninvited "twisted sisters" as an object lesson.

By this time in my life, I was not working out—or, more to the point, I did not really know how to work out in a gym—and scuba diving and other physical stimuli were not happening as frequently as before, so my right side, with

CP, started to become weaker and weaker by the day, to the point of greatly affecting my health. I did not yet understand the concept of "use it or lose it," and my stronger left side had been pulling double to triple duty for my weaker right side for many years. Stress was building up on my left, especially in my back and neck, and the strain was becoming unbearable—something was about to give.

THE MIAMI BUST

In 2001, I decided to leave the corporate world for a while to return to graduate school due to my love of learning and the "newness" that surrounds school life. This had always been my intention since leaving formal undergraduate learning in 1993.

On a graduate school scouting trip to Miami, Florida, in early January 2003, I herniated two disks in my neck while sleeping on an oversized pillow. I thought it was the result of a one-time event from sleeping wrong on a hard pillow, but I later learned it was due to a systemic buildup of stress in my neck muscles. Years of job-related stress, lack of exercise, lack of balanced core, and weak right-side muscle tone due to my CP had led to this bust. Basically, my left side could no longer support what my right side should have been doing all along. The stress accumulated in my neck because my left side was doing more work than it was supposed to have ever done. My right side was not able to balance the load, and my neck became the focal point for a disaster years in the making. I had even started seeing a chiropractor in the 1990s to help relieve tension and pain and to put my body back into alignment. Like I was made of LEGOs, my chiropractor could put me back into alignment, but due to my lack of right-side muscle tone and functioning, the LEGOs always fell apart again.

Crazy things were happening to my body, and I knew only of the symptoms. When my disks "snapped" on January 17, 2003, I had intense pain in my neck. My right arm was almost completely numb from my fingertips to my shoulder, and my right forearm bone marrow felt like it was freezing (don't ask me how I know what freezing bone marrow feels like). I was losing hope of long-term relief.

After I herniated my disks, I spent the following day in the Miami-Dade County ER, where they assessed my situation, took low-tech X-rays, and sent me on my way with a prescription of ibuprofen, even though I had trouble breathing due to the intense pain.

Before I returned on an emergency flight back to Austin to see my own doctor, I decided that I should contact the University of Miami and apologize for missing our planned interview appointment and ask to reschedule my visit before I returned home. The irony of this situation was that I ended up meeting Dr. Joel Stutz, the dean of the business school's computer information systems program, in a neck brace, in pain, and ended that long day with his high recommendation of unconditional acceptance to his program at the University of Miami as a graduate student for the 2003 term—a school I would have never applied to or been accepted to had it not been for this last-minute, unplanned, painful visit with Dr. Stutz. After all, I was scheduled to return home without visiting the school at all.

I ended up attending graduate school from 2003 to 2005 at the University of Miami and graduated with a master of science in computer information systems, in high standing.

THIS CUP OF SUFFERING

Upon my return to Austin, I went to a doctor who specialized in neck disorders like mine. After a series of high-tech X-rays and MRIs, he diagnosed me with a large dorsolateral disk herniation at C6 and C7 and a small left disk dorsolateral disk herniation at C5 and C6. The disk on my right side was pressing against the nerve root that went down my right arm, causing major pain and numbness throughout my right shoulder, down to my right hand and fingers, including my shoulder blade and lower neck. Surprisingly, there were no discernible symptoms on my left side from C5 to C6, even though the nerve root was affected by the herniation. My doctor recommended I undergo an operation called anterior cervical diskectomy and fusion with instrumentation to remove the ruptured disks and fuse C6 and C7, and C5 and C6 together. A radical operation, in my book. He prescribed a selective nerve-root block at C6 and C7, a script for hydrocodone—a strong narcotic painkiller that made me drool and sleep a lot—and a cervical neck brace in the meantime. I sought out two other doctors to confirm or deny his diagnosis. To my dismay, both confirmed that I needed the surgery. I prayed for relief from the intense pain I was going through, hoped for a miracle, and began to listen to His guidance.

Four days before my pending surgery, I was driving across town, running errands before my life-altering surgery was to be performed. I'd had an unbelievably bad premonition about this upcoming procedure from day one, but the doctors knew best. Or so I thought. On a whim, I decided to stop by Austin Aqua Sports, one of my favorite scuba dive shops that I'd spent a lot of time in prior to all this mess. The store was located at the corner of Forty-Fifth and Guadalupe Street, a location that was not on my normal path for that day. I knew the owner and manager well, and I decided to stop in and let them know about my trip to Florida, about the dives I had planned, and about my neck issue. After all, I had planned to dive in Florida with my rebreather while I was out there, but all that changed in a "snap." Seems that fate was starting to show that very day.

Mike Nickell, who looked very much like Kenny Rogers, was the owner of Austin Aqua Sports. I talked about my trip to Florida and my doctor's prognosis; he was genuinely concerned. "Under no circumstances let this doctor operate on you," he said. "Wait right here." Then he quickly departed the room. Perplexed, I waited for his return. I could hear him rummaging around in the back room for something, although I knew not what.

Then he returned. "I cannot tell you why; however, *do not* let this doctor operate on you," he reiterated. "Call this doctor in Houston and schedule an appointment with him right away," he said as he handed me the doctor's card. He insisted I call right then. I reached for my cell phone and, as best I could, held it up to my left ear without moving my neck. I called and scheduled an appointment for the very next day, after they learned how close I was to my operation date.

Driving to Houston from Austin was a very painful and long drive. But it's a drive that I am incredibly grateful I took. The doctor in Houston took a look at my "antiquated" MRI film that I'd brought with me and ordered another round of MRI scans to be sure of his recommendation. While the technologist was scanning me, he wanted to confirm that I had CP. I thought this was a weird question, but I was in too much pain to really care; all I said was, "Yes, I do."

He looked back at the scans on his monitor again and said, "Your brain scans look great. There is no trace of brain damage at all." He continued to say that he would have doubted I had cerebral palsy at all from what he saw on my MRI brain scans.

I was amazed because, up to this point in my life, I had always been told that once the brain was damaged, it's not repairable, something I learned when I was a small kid. Doctors had told my parents that the brain was hardwired, and once damaged, it's not reversible.[32] This new information from Houston ultimately led to me to begin my research into neuroplasticity.

"I'm not saying you don't require an operation. However, let's put this off and try a less invasive procedure and see if we can get these disks back into place so they can heal. First of all, let's get you off these narcotics so you can think clearly," my new doctor said.

My new doctor was recommending three things: The first was a nonnarcotic painkiller that was not opiate-based or habit-forming. The second was traction to increase the spaces between my vertebrae. The third was physical therapy using the McKenzie protocol to realign the disks and strengthen my neck support muscles to allow the disks to regenerate. I was ecstatic. I was thrilled. It was as if a weight had been literally lifted from me that day.

I then made two other phone calls. One, to cancel my operation three days out, and two, to my family to let them know there was hope once again.

It took around nine months for the numbness in my right arm to fully decentralize (recede) and disappear and the disks in my neck to miraculously regenerate. Lots of outpatient physical therapy (PT), cervical traction, and lots of homework utilizing the McKenzie Protocol. No permanent damage, no long-term health problems…just a reminder that I had come within three days of a life-altering operation that would have shortened my stature by two or so inches and ended my scuba diving career at best and possibly much, much worse consequences. By the time graduate school at the University of Miami began, I was fully healed.

A year later, Mike Nickell and his wife, Cat, along with other folks from Austin Aqua Sports, came to the Florida Keys to dive with me. We spent a wonderful weekend of diving wrecks and reefs in the Keys as well as attending the Diving Equipment and Marketing Association expo in Miami (for dive retailers, leaders, and instructors in the scuba diving industry). In the evenings, we sat on the dock on the Gulf side of the Keys, reminiscing about good old times while watching the sun set over Texas, far out in the Gulf of Mexico. Mike then told me the rest of the story of why he had passionately persuaded me to forgo my originally scheduled operation. Mike was a retired doctor himself and was in litigation as an expert witness against my would-be surgeon at the time of my visit. Since the case was in litigation, he could not talk about it at that time. However, the case had since been won and settled, and he could now discuss the findings. The court case was for the same surgery I was going to have with the same doctor. Mike had been called as an expert medical witness for the prosecution, representing a patient who ended up a quadriplegic from this doctor's procedure. It was determined that this doctor had performed a botched, unapproved procedure, which was an unnecessary operation altogether, only to benefit this doctor's medical status and research. Apparently, my friend had recognized the shocking similarities with my case and the lawsuit he was involved in and did not want me to fall into the same trap. I was very grateful. God had removed this cup from me and protected me from more harm. I ended up buying the next several rounds of drinks with gratitude.

SCUBA DIVING IN THE KEYS

Nearly twenty years after my Rescue Diver class, I was in the Florida Keys during my time at the University of Miami (2003 to 2005). To be exact, I was in Key Largo, on dive location. A seasoned, salty seafaring Captain Spencer Slate, owner of Atlantis Dive Center, and I were sitting on the bridge of the *Star Fish*, one of the dive boats in his fleet. We were talking about his various diving adventures while students from the University of Miami Scuba Club were bubbling far below on the USS *Spiegel Grove* wreck. I decided to sit out this dive to warm up and enjoy another fine afternoon out at sea.

Slate and I had become friends over the last two years while I was in graduate school. During this time, I served on the University of Miami Scuba Club as a board member and as a liaison to all the local dive shop operators up and down the Florida Keys and most of South Florida. I enjoyed hanging out on his boats in the stillness of the moment, watching all the happenings on board and assisting as a divemaster and fellow diver. Captain Slate asked me if I had ever wanted to go for my Instructor rating. After all, he said, he had seen me bring down nearly four hundred students to his shop over the last two years, and he knew how competent a technical diver I was. He also mentioned that I was particularly good at keeping these guys from UM in line and was an excellent officer and liaison. Week after week, I would book slots with his office manager, Lena "Bean" Scott-Loveday, and each week, I got out and enjoyed the splendor of the underwater world of the Keys. I was even part of Tom and Lena's underwater wedding, with Captain Slate officiating in a bunny costume, which ended up in the Guinness World Records book: "The largest underwater wedding took place on 31 October 2004 when a record 110 scuba divers submerged to the City of Washington wreck, Elbow Reef off the coast of Florida Keys, USA, to witness the marriage ceremony between Lena Scott and Tom Loveday (both USA)."

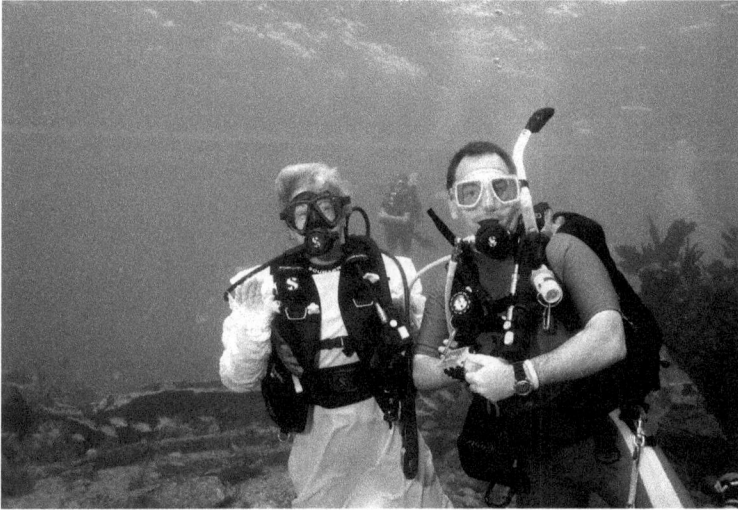

With Lena Loveday at her wedding to Tom

My response to Captain Slate was that, no, I had never thought of continuing my education to become an instructor. He then mentioned that my prep work for my Instructor Development Course (IDC)—diver evaluations and skills checkout—would be waived due to the high level of competency and rich diving résumé he and his other instructors had already witnessed and experienced with me. After all, not only had I gone diving with him and the University of Miami Scuba Club, but I also dove my Dräger rebreather with other technical divers and his crew. He said I was a natural at this stuff and I would be that much more ahead if I decided to pursue my Instructor rating. I was intrigued and continued to ask more questions, gathering intel while out at sea that day.

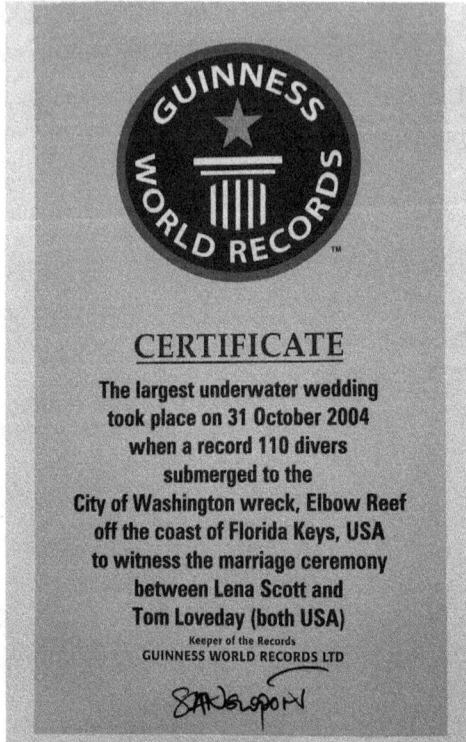

Participant at the Guinness World Record underwater wedding

After I completed the IDC training program in the Keys on February 5, 2005, Captain Spencer Slate presented me as a new National Association of Underwater Instructors (NAUI) scuba instructor. A special note to this achievement is that my final IDC dive completion check was signed off by my good friend and dive mentor Tom McCoy, now working for NASA at their underwater buoyancy lab in Houston, Texas. Tom was there as one of my Open Water instructors at the very beginning back in 1986, and I was honored that he was there to sign off on the very last requirement of my IDC Instructor training. I envisioned that Jacques Cousteau would've been proud of me that day.

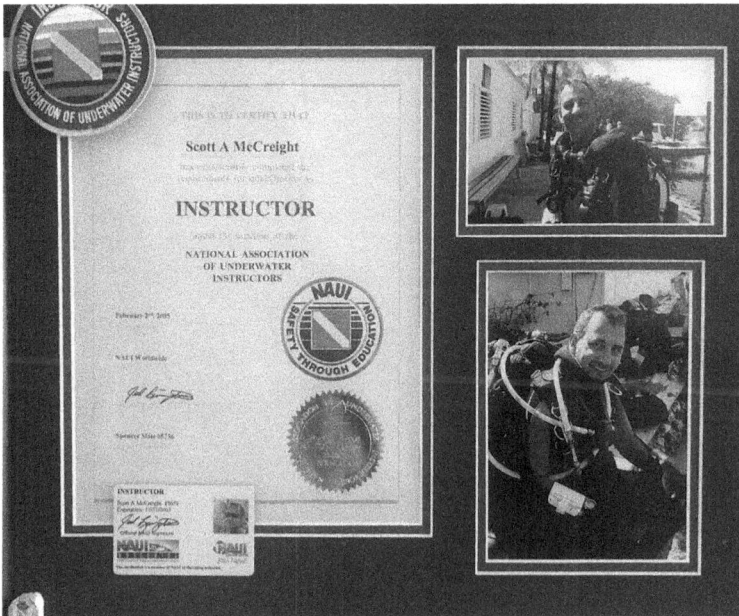

My framed Instructor rating 2003

As of today, I have over eight hundred hours underwater, have traveled to exotic scuba diving locations all over the world, and have more than eighteen certifications, including technical mixed gas (heliox) for very deep saturation diving, passive SCR and active SCR rebreather, and cave diving.

All of this happened because of a dream that a fifteen-year-old kid with cerebral palsy had and was encouraged to follow through on. Building new skills, experiences, and, best of all, confidence to overcome the "impossible" was the key I needed to succeed. Faith and encouragement from others will always inspire the human potential to reach way beyond perceived "limits."

Leo and Extreme Sports

IT SEEMED THAT I HAD DEVELOPED A PROPENSITY FOR AND CONTINUED to gravitate toward extreme, technically challenging sports like scuba diving and skydiving, as was the case in high school and college. As I climbed the scuba certification ladder early in life, I realized that I loved learning challenging sports that were highly technical and "life-threatening." Those sports that, for the most part, others would never be able to do or were not willing to try, I wanted to experience and even master. My CP drove me even harder to achieve something that "they" could not or would not do.

If the playing field had been level for me like it was for others, I would have been able to compete in "regular sports." However, in the case of these extreme, technically challenging activities such as scuba diving, it was not a level field. It was a highly technical, "mentally intense" field. And I competed with myself for mastery.

In the case of scuba diving, I went in two different directions. I became an instructor with NAUI after going through Open Water, Advanced Open Water, Rescue, Master Diver, and Divemaster with PADI, as mentioned earlier. However, I also became a highly technical master diver by going deep into the technical side of scuba diving. This includes work from the International Association of Nitrox and Technical Divers with certifications in

Nitrox, Advanced Nitrox, Dräger Atlantis Rebreather Diver, and Advanced Trimix. I also certified with Technical Diving International for Dräger Dolphin Rebreather, Cavern Diver, and Cave Diver, along with Specialty Deep Diver, and Equipment Specialist certifications with PADI. And with Scuba Schools International, I am also certified on the Mares/rEvo Horizon - Rebreather.

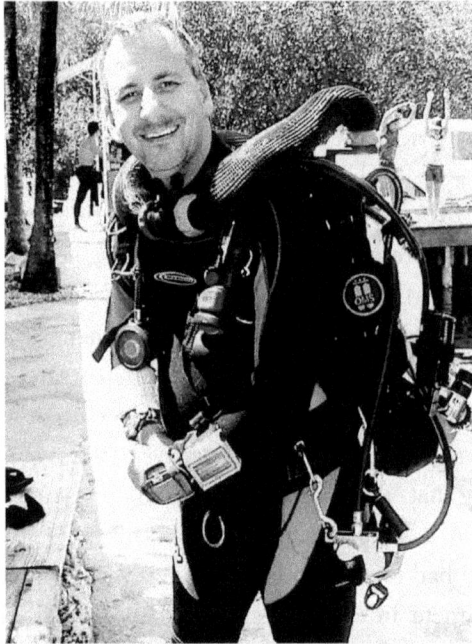

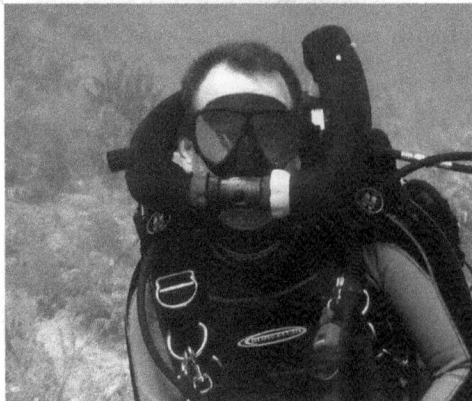

Scott and his rebreather scuba gear

LIFE-SUPPORT LEARNING

I love learning challenging activities that require advanced life-support equipment and learning advanced mental and physical skills to survive and thrive in an otherwise hostile or deadly environment. Sports such as skydiving and scuba diving, rappelling, and skiing are exciting sports I have fallen in love with. I wonder if this is not the result of all that life-support gear I was hooked up to as a preemie baby so long ago. It seemed that Leo had mastered the world around him, and little baby Frankenstein was now into technical life-support sports.

Mixed-gas diving, such as deep trimix diving and cave diving, is quite gear intensive and requires many hours of mental training and skill mastering along with staying physically fit. This type of scuba diving is not for the faint of heart. Over many years, I met and learned from the absolute best in the industry. Scuba legends like Richard Rydell, James Bowden, Sheck Exley, Al Pertner, Paul Murphy and Tanya Streeter, to name just a few, taught me not only how to survive underwater but also to thrive and grow in confidence and keep challenging myself to learn and explore more. I even took several of my friends along with me on these journeys. These great divers became friends over the years, and what they taught me, in some cases, came directly from actual postmortems from dive fatalities …a fact that still haunts me at every dive briefing.

CAVE DIVING—HOW I FELL INTO A HOLE AND SURVIVED

"Hey! Let's fall into a small water hole in the ground and spend hours in cold, watery pitch-blackness, carrying all our breathing gas through tiny, cramped openings with only a small string to follow!" This is not something that you simply wake up one day and say. A more accurate assessment is that a group of diving friends invited me to partake in the adventure of a lifetime down on the Yucatán Peninsula in Central America. *What an adventure it would be!* I thought. I would be trained in three of the four cave diving certifications by a specialized team of cave divers in a three-week intensive course all set up for us. How could I pass up the opportunity?

Al Pertner was our cave instructor with Akumal Dive Shop, out of the tiny village of Akumal, Mexico. Our training started on dry land with lots of cave diving theory and practice laying line. This line work, or what we later called "string theory," was critical to master on land before entering the dark underwater world. Our lives would literally depend upon this line work! The string would be our lifeline back into the light. As we entered the cave, we would run a line with us so that when we "turned the dive" (turned around to return to our starting point—the daylight), we could follow the line back out. Sounds simple, right? Try doing this blindfolded in a cave. To practice this skill in the water, we placed duct tape over our masks. Then, to make things even harder and more unexpected, we removed one fin, or had no mask on at all, or used a buddy's air supply, simulating various types of emergencies. We learned that this was *not* so simple. The instructors drilled these skills into us as we practiced in a confined body of water over and over under timed trials. Over and over. We also simulated scenarios such as running out of breathing gas, encountering a panicked diver or an unconscious diver, and so on. Over and over, day after day, we practiced these drills. After all, as I said before, complacency kills, and underwater in caves, complacency will sneak up on you fast.

The big day came—first a cavern dive in the morning to practice what we had done on land or in a confined body of water just days before. After the cavern dive, we debriefed and then planned and progressed to diving our very first cave. What a blast! I was actually doing the stuff that I'd watched on the National Geographic channel just weeks ago.

In diving, a cavern is defined as an overhang, with no direct ascent possible to the surface but still within the daylight zone, whereas a cave is defined as having no light from above and no ascent to the surface without egress to the cavern zone.

We dove several famous cenotes (underground cave systems) over a three-week period around Tulum and Akumal—caves such as Car Wash, Dos Ojos, Tajma Ha, Garden of Eden/Ponderosa, to name a few. I was so stoked that I was being trained to dive in places that only National Geographic film teams would go with "real" cave divers. I was in training to be one of these guys. I was truly blessed to have experienced and been trained by these dive legends.

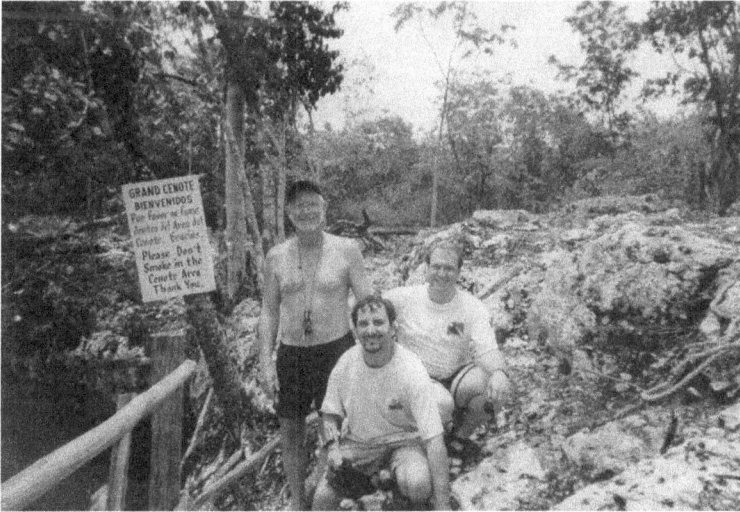

Scott and his team, cave diving in Akumal, Mexico

MIXING IT UP A BIT

Mixed-gas diving is another very advanced scuba training program that I dove into, and like cave diving, it essentially dropped into my lap. While in Florida in graduate school, I was introduced to Richard Rydell while serving on the Miami Scuba Club board (2003 to 2005).[33] Richard and I quickly became good friends because of our shared love of scuba diving. Richard was impressed with my vast background in technical diving and offered me an opportunity of a lifetime…an opportunity to go deep, and I mean really deep, diving with a training program called Accelerated Decompression Scuba Diving. This would require special training, exotic blends of breathing gas, and special equipment, most of which I surprisingly already had on hand. I would be learning about and totally dependent on breathing a hypoxic (less than 21 percent oxygen) gas mixture called trimix and heliox at 350 feet underwater in the Florida Keys.

Trimix is a breathing gas consisting of oxygen, helium, and nitrogen. This mixture is unique to the depth in which a diver will descend and is often used in deep diving, whereas heliox is typically a mixture of less than 21 percent oxygen and the rest helium, for very deep saturation diving. During the deep phase of the dive, divers switch to this gas. Even though the concentration of oxygen is below 21 percent, this mixture is not hypoxic at these depths due to the nature of gas physics and partial pressure of oxygen on our nervous system to support life. Heliox breathing gases are for very technical and advanced diving and not used for recreational scuba diving.

Helium is included as an inert gas taking the place of some, if not all, of the nitrogen to reduce the dangerous narcotic effects of nitrogen gas at great depths. With a mixture of three gases, it is possible to create exotic mixes suitable for different depths by adjusting the proportions of each gas. Oxygen content can be optimized for the depth to limit the risk of oxygen toxicity (a.k.a. central nervous system toxicity) by lowering the total amount of oxygen below the 21 percent (hypoxic) threshold we breathe on land (at sea level). If we were to breathe less than 21 percent oxygen on land (at sea level) under heavy stress, we would pass out due to hypoxia. However, under these tremendous pressures and stressors underwater, the reduced amount of oxygen is life-sustaining. The remaining two inert gas components are balanced between nitrogen and helium. By increasing the level of helium, which is not narcotic at these depths like nitrogen is, the diver is able to remain conscious and fully alert. Helium is also a smaller molecule, which, under these pressures, allows for a significant reduction in a diver's work of breathing, due to helium not causing excess molecular friction during the breathing process.

I had to learn lots of advanced life-support theory and cool stuff like advanced physics, chemistry, and human physiology to stay alive and function under all that water. But I ate this material up like cereal for breakfast. I loved those "scuba snacks," as we called them, a direct reference to Scooby-Doo's Scooby Snacks. It was as if I was made for this stuff.

Richard and I dove many decompression-type deep dives in the Florida Keys, such as to the USCGC *Bibb*, which was named after the secretary of the Treasury under President John Tyler and was built in 1936 as part of a group of seven ships, including the USCGC *Duane*. What an awesome dive! The *Bibb* lies on its starboard (right) side in hard running water (currents). We also dove the USS *Spiegel Grove* (LSD-32), 510 feet long and 84 feet wide, located on Dixie Shoal, six miles off the Keys in the Florida Keys National Marine Sanctuary.[34] She was sunk on June 10, 2002 and had come to rest on her port (left) side when we dove it. However, Hurricane Dennis turned the ship upright in July 2005, years after I had left the Keys.

These deep dives were amazing. We carried twin 85 tanks on our backs and two smaller tanks side-mounted under each arm. Each tank has a different mixture of gas in it and is attached to an independent regulator to breathe from. At a predefined depth, we would switch breathing gases and descend deeper. At a predetermined time and depth, we would inflate a lift bag with a line similar to our cave lines and slowly ascend in what is known as an accelerated decompression dive procedure. By switching to a higher level of oxygen/helium mixture (low nitrogen) while ascending and hanging out at predetermined depths and times, I was able to remove the accumulated nitrogen from my body, significantly reducing the possibility of getting the bends. This ascent would usually last for fifteen to twenty-five minutes, with a stop at fifteen feet for two minutes or more on 100 percent oxygen to remove as much nitrogen from my body as possible. This always felt like a long time to ascend. Needless to say, on each dive, we had to know exactly which regulator to breathe from at each portion of the dive, or we would be in trouble for sure. After all, we would not want to breathe 100 percent oxygen at 130 feet.

A TWENTY-FIRST-CENTURY
THREE-HOUR TOUR

One of my deep dives was particularly challenging, and I had to rely on all of my experience and training to survive it. This dive was in very rough seas—with fifteen-foot swells and a strong surface current. I dove in with my four tanks before Jon Boley, my dive buddy. I followed the downline with Jon in tow, fighting the waves and current most of the way. When I made it to the wreck, at 350 feet, Jon was not behind me. He had been right behind me when we left the surface. *Where in the heck did he go?* I thought. Richard held up two fingers right next to one another, signaling, *Where is your buddy?* I looked around, then Richard signaled me to turn the dive in order to find my buddy. Now, I can't just come straight up from 350 feet down breathing trimix with an oxygen level well below 21 percent, or I would get the bends, pass out, and drown. I had to follow my training, emergency procedures, and dive plan. I deployed my lift bag (with my name on it so the dive boat knew who was on the way up). I started my solo ascent, following my gas management plan and predetermined gas switches. For twenty-eight minutes of decompression, I ascended slowly and stopped at predetermined stops per plan. I kept wondering about Jon. *Was he okay? Was the boat going to be there when I surfaced?* Controlling your mind on deep dives like this is a matter of life or death. No time for me to panic. *Scott, get a hold of yourself. Rely on your training, and focus on the plan*, I thought.

Up I went, switching breathing gas (regulators) at my preset switch points as the current dragged me here and there. The upline with lift bag kept me at the right depth. After what seemed like an eternity, I surfaced. The dive boat was there, waiting for me. I gave the "okay" symbol by forming a big O with my arms on the top of my head while keeping my regulator in my mouth. The waves were now fifteen to twenty feet high, and strong winds and stormy skies created whitecaps. It took the divemasters another fifteen minutes to successfully throw me a pickup "tow line" and haul me in after three failed attempts—very rough and crazy seas. It reminded me of the intro to *Gilligan's Island*, and the theme song kept poking its way into my consciousness.

After I was hauled into the boat by tow line, I then detached each of my side-mounted decompression tanks and handed them up to the divemaster, one by one, taking another fifteen minutes to hand up all my auxiliary tech gear. Then I clipped my fins to my buoyancy compensator and climbed the twelve-rung ladder with only my twin back scuba tanks and my OMS tech-pack BC on my back as the boat heaved up and down. A mere one hundred pounds of gear plus my body weight to lift while the boat pitched to and fro. Up the ladder I went with each wave. Up, up I went. I hit the dive deck, and while the deck support divemasters were helping me remove my tech gear, there sat Jon, looking like a drowned rat.

We were glad to see each other. I asked, "What happened down there?"

He said that his main regulator started to free-flow uncontrollably, and he had to abort the dive. He only made it down fifty feet or so before turning back. I was not within reach, so he could not signal me. I sure was glad he was okay. I was also glad that all my training had kicked in and I made it back safely without incident.

Upon our official dive debrief, Richard commended me for an excellent unplanned emergency abort and follow-through. He said, "This is even more proof that this young man with CP can hang with the very best of the technical diver community."

This was my final dive certifying me as an Advanced Trimix Deep Diver with technical honors. I had mastered some of the most challenging, life-threatening dive obstacles on this one dive alone, what seemed like a twenty-first-century version of a *Gilligan's Island* "three-hour tour" boat ride—and all with CP.

I added rebreather diving (the air a diver breathes out is recirculated, scrubbing the carbon dioxide out and adding in oxygen and a dilutant called breathing gas as needed) to my dive résumé in the same way—the opportunity just seemed to present itself to me through an instructor, and once I was on closed-circuit rebreather gear, my world of scuba diving was about to change forever. Quiet, very few bubbles, and so relaxing. No noise other than your breathing and the clicking of one-way-breathing valves. It's just you and the sea, or in my first experience, a pool with fish painted on the sides and coral painted on the bottom.

As part of my certification, I bought my first rebreather, a Dräger Dolphin semi-closed-circuit rebreather, and I made several trips with this rig to places like Bonaire and Cozumel. Soon after, I modified it to be a closed-circuit rebreather. Add in mixed-gas mixtures to closed and semi-closed-circuit rebreather diving, and I was loving every minute underwater, no matter the exotic dive location. This is the way to dive!

As I mentioned earlier, in the Introduction, a friend once told me that I don't do easy well—but damn, I do hard very well. Upon reflection, I think this may be quite true. As a shy kid with many early failures in life, I must have subconsciously decided that on a "level playing field," I would not be able to "do simple" very well and therefore did not want to play that game. Instead, I found challenging sports such as these that were demanding, challenging, and seemed hard by able-bodied standards. They required a lot of technical training that most people would never even attempt.

Extreme sports such as cave, deep mixed gas, and rebreather diving (to name a few), as well as NAUI Instructor certification, all take tremendous amounts of training, mental discipline, and physical stamina to successfully master. When I started diving at the age of sixteen, I had no idea that I would go on to master these ambitious sport activities—after all, people said I could not do all that with CP. Don't *ever* tell a child with CP he or she can't do _____ (fill in the blank) because of CP. I recommend that we turn that statement into "I can't do that…yet!"

A good friend once told me, "It's simply amazing and inspirational that you are doing all of these things with CP. Most able-bodied people will never dare attempt to do half of what you have already overcome in life. We can't wait to see what is next."

This same wisdom should apply to all of us, regardless of our (dis)abilities. We all need to remember to think positively and remind ourselves that it's not that we can't do it. *We can't do it…yet.*

Leo was about to learn just how many things he could really do, even though he'd been told he could never do them. Leo was about to bloom!

PART 5

Putting My Brain in My Locker

Mice Can Move Elephants

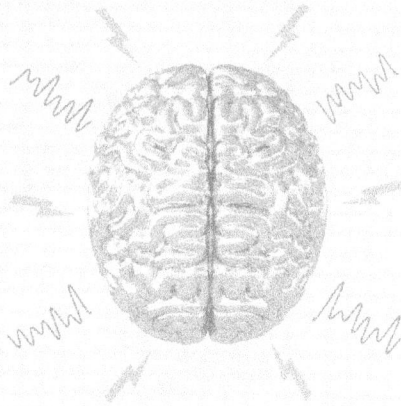

My First
Personal Trainer

FAST-FORWARD TO THE FALL OF 2011. I WAS UNDEREMPLOYED, working for a startup company—and little did I know by this time in my life, I was extremely out of shape because complacency had taken over. My father and stepmother had been working out with help from a personal trainer at one of the Gold's Gyms in South Austin for close to a year. Both seemed to be having a great time decreasing their body size, bettering their physique, "complaining" about all the aches and pains that go along with working out, and really enjoying improving their bodies with this trainer. It was exciting listening to them talk about their workout sessions week after week and about how their trainer would make them do this and do that. My stepmother's stories of their workouts and incurring pain at the hands of this trainer were intriguing to say the least. The trainer not only kept my champion water-skiing dad in tip-top shape but also kept my stepmother and dad fully engaged with fitness.

Around Christmastime, Dad asked me what I wanted for Christmas. After thinking long and hard, I said, "I really don't want anything other than maybe a gym membership and a couple hours with a trainer to learn how to work out without 'killing' myself." Besides, I really wanted to meet this person who was training my father and stepmother and actually getting away with it.

To my great surprise, Dad gave me a gift that would end up changing the trajectory of my life. This gift, coupled with determination, hard work, and a newly discovered drive for excellence, would also change a lot of other lives in the days to follow…but I am getting way ahead of myself again.

That Christmas, a Gold's Gym membership and a few sessions with one of their top trainers was mine to claim. As part of my gift, Dad asked who I wanted as a trainer out of all the trainers on their staff. "I want your trainer," I replied. "I want to be trained by Ruth King." As I said, I wanted to meet their famous trainer.

UNIQUE WORKOUT SESSIONS

My first experience walking into Gold's wasn't a typical one. It was one of their older South Austin locations, off Ben White Boulevard, near what used to be the old Southwood Theater, where I'd seen *Star Trek* as a preteen many years ago. I had not been to that part of town in years. The gym, known as South Central, was equipped with a track and lots of intimidating workout equipment. No tour, no sales pitch, no "easing the client into working out and making him feel good." Oh no, it was straight to the workout floor for me, and an all-too-familiar phrase soon followed: "Give me a lap."

My first session and quite a few after that were very basic. No weights, no rest, no waiting to catch my breath or even ask questions. Ruth just had me perform simple alignment and stability work, which I would later learn was called "core development." Memories of the Austin CP Center kept creeping back into my consciousness. I had not tripped into these recessed memories in a long, long time. I had for years kept repressing these thoughts into the black abyss of my mind, trying to become normal. After all, I was now a grown adult and thought I had done so much improving since those early days.

Ruth would snap me back into the moment. "Focus, Scott!" Then she would have me run another lap. I think she called this phase of training "baseline skill devolvement and measurements."

These first sessions consisted of nothing more than "proper" sitting, then sitting to standing, and lying on stability balls at all sorts of different positions and angles, as well as elbow planks and walking on a treadmill just like my old days at the CP Center. Part of me kept looking around for my old friend, that big, round, colorful ball. The treadmill was the hardest part. People with hemiplegia or lower diplegia cerebral palsy don't typically have a "normal" walking gait. For me, this meant I was walking on my right toes with my right foot turning out as opposed to the correct flat and stable straight foot, heel-toe, heel-toe stepping movement. I would also lean to my left side as I walked, causing a hip imbalance, which led to spine misalignment. Nothing seemed to escape Ruth's eye for physical training perfection.

About two weeks into our sessions, Ruth took me aside and apologized for the way she had begun our training together. "I've known about you for over a year now, through your father and stepmother, and I was so excited to get to work with you," she said. "Your father has talked about you so much, and I really wanted to meet you. I realize you don't know anything about me. I took this for granted and put you straight to work."

I smiled a bit and chuckled. After all, this was one of the few times somebody did not automatically treat me with kid gloves with respect to my CP. She did not give me the "You can't do that, so why bother" attitude toward what I could accomplish on the workout floor. Usually I had to "prove" to others, through determination and sheer resolve, that I was worthy. But here in *her* gym, Ruth immediately put me to task, solving difficulties that I've had my entire life, most of which I never knew I had, and I learned more with each session.

It seemed I was now ending the period of my life marked by denial and avoidance. It was time to learn how to fight and remove complacency entirely from my life.

Ruth also told me that, for whatever reason, I had subconsciously learned that "I could not do this" or "I could not do that." She said this was a flat-out lie and set out to prove it. She was going to change the paradigm on what I thought I could accomplish as a new athlete. She was not only going to teach my body how to build muscles, but she was also going to teach me to "fight" for what I was able to do and not automatically "flee" from the challenges she would soon put me through. I was no longer allowed to say the following three words on *her* workout floor: *can't, try,* and *no.* Words that conveyed failure. Words that subconsciously signaled that I had already given up. And before this point, I tended to say those words a lot.

As the weeks progressed, Ruth introduced me to small, thin, round rubber bands with handles. Then I moved on to big, thick rubber bands and gradually stepped up to "typical" workout equipment. In those early days, she would modify the angles of my pulls and pushes by adding straps and tying me down to various cable machines to get my weak right arm and leg to move properly. It was extremely frustrating and, at the same time, so much fun to learn these new techniques. Frustrating in that my body did not yet know how to properly perform these movements (because of incorrect muscle memory) and fun because I wanted to learn all I could about why we were doing what we were doing (novelty). To say that I was always curious was an understatement.

At the gym, it became routine to see me tied up to a cable row or cable lat-pull machine. Ruth would tie my left hand behind my back to get my right shoulder and arm to pull correctly since my right hand was not yet capable of gripping handles and my right wrist was not strong or straight enough to engage properly. Ruth would routinely inform her general manager, "Scott is coming in today," so that if her staff received "complaints" about one of their trainers tying up clients on the workout floor, she would know that it was just Ruth working with me. Her general manager had quite a laugh about the various *complaints* that other members expressed due to Ruth's atypical training style.

This atypical training style was not lost on onlookers alone. For instance, one of my favorite routines included performing an elbow plank on a medicine ball with the added difficulty of her kneeling on top of me. Yes, Ruth convinced me that I was strong enough to not only perform a plank on an unstable platform but to do so while supporting her entire body weight on top of me. I ate this up and thought it was so cool that I was now not only able to perform a plank on a medicine ball—that was hard enough—but to amp it up a notch (or three) by having Ruth kneel on top of me. Reviewing the filmed routines was a real motivator for me and a very novel approach to training.

During another workout session, Ruth had me put on a brand-new Gold's Challenge shirt. Then she took a pair of scissors and began to cut the arms off (while I was still in the shirt), transforming it into my first ever "muscle shirt." She said this would allow me to see my muscles engage while we were in session. As she cut the arms off, other patrons began to gather. I was still shy but secretly enjoyed all the positive attention. Her plan worked brilliantly. As the weeks progressed, I wore that shirt proudly to every session like a new badge of honor, watching my new muscles grow. Even today, every time I put on that muscle shirt, I can't help but smile at the way this one act changed the image of that shy young man in the lobby of her gym.

Ruth's novel approach to solving difficult problems did not end there.

CURIOSITY DID NOT KILL THE MOUSE

I have always been—and was subsequently trained to be—an analytical thinker. I am an engineer, and growing up shy and introverted naturally led me down this path. Ruth would constantly tell me to not ask any questions and that she would explain later…much later, if at all. She would simply tell me to go *put my brain in my locker* and just do what she wanted me to do. At first, I thought she was telling me this as a defense mechanism that a trainer would employ to get the trainee to perform (trainee stall tactic, perhaps), and it ticked me off because I wanted to learn. I wanted to understand what was really going on.

My engineering background and inquisitive nature have compelled me to always analyze everything: how to improve this or that in everything I do. As an industrial systems engineer, it's all about efficiency. It's our goal to redesign the machine to fit "man's needs." It was ingrained in me to want to redesign the system I was in front of to accommodate me, or rather, the old me. However, this was not the purpose of the machines and systems in the gym. The purpose of these machines was to allow me to function and move properly to build muscles. Apparently, my brain was getting in the way of her work, subconsciously sabotaging her efforts to get my body to do what it was not yet aware it could do. By "putting my brain in my locker," I painfully learned to turn off my analytical mind, to do what I needed to do on her workout floor. If only she had communicated her intentions up front, this would have made the start of my transformation a lot smoother for the both of us.

Another way of looking at this is to think of a mouse. When setting up a stimulus-response experiment, where you watch a mouse run in a maze or analyze the behavior of that mouse while he runs to or from known stimuli, you typically do not tell the mouse what you are doing or what you expect him to do. That would change the outcome of the experiment, if the mouse could understand what was going on in the first place (perhaps a bit of foreshadowing). In my case, Ruth was experimenting, learning what my "triggers" were to known stressors and observing the reactions of my body. She wanted me to "turn off my analytical brain" and just do what she instructed. By putting my brain in my locker, she was able to work with my body without me, or rather my mind, getting in her way. Leo had transformed into a gym mouse. I was learning how to work her *maze* without my mind subconsciously sabotaging her work.

I found it both intriguing and exciting that I was beginning to use my right side properly and starting to feel the burn of brand-new muscles developing, some for the first time ever. Needless to say, her unique approaches to this transformation were not entirely lost in my locker, and I secretly liked boasting to my buddies that I was being tied up by my female trainer on her workout floor. As an added bonus, the videos of her kneeling on me while I held a plank for a minute plus on a medicine ball were just the proof I needed to convince my subconscious of what I was now capable of doing.

This novel transformation was simply amazing, and I desired to achieve even more.

GIVE ME A LAP

The first gym that Ruth and I started training at had a three-lane track in the middle of it. Each lap was one-thirteenth of a mile or approximately 123 meters.

Early on in our training sessions, Ruth noticed a negative pattern in my think-ing that she needed to break quickly if we were ever going to see any positive results. At the beginning, I was overcome with fear inside the gym, like a timid mouse. Not so much emotional external fear, but internal (for the most part) subconscious fear. I don't know if this originated from repressed, buried memories from school PE classes or from a lack of confidence within any gym environment up to this point, but nevertheless, the fear was strong enough to negatively affect my body.

From a kinesiology perspective, in our bodies, sympathetic nerves only have two responses, "flight" or "fight." And Ruth knew that she needed to find my "trigger" to get my brain to listen to her training and not to my own subcon-scious fear. In theory, running would shock my system and overload my brain so it wouldn't have time to think about what I was doing and would instead just do it. Ruth identified this as my trigger. Up to this point, there had not been a significant amount of research done to prove whether this working theory would be beneficial in adults with CP, but she was willing to give it a go. She would employ anything to get me out of my own head, so to speak.

So, during our early set of sessions, she put her theory to the test without me, the timid mouse, ever knowing. "Scott, give me a lap around the track as fast as you can run," she would tell me whenever she noticed this negative pattern emerging.

These sessions were like no other workouts I had known. And bam, they worked like a charm. At every lap, as she timed me, she would yell, "Faster, faster, Scott. You can do this!"

I wanted to please my trainer so badly that I would fight to run faster every time.

Yes! I can *do this,* I would think to myself. Subconsciously, I no longer thought of what actual difficulties I was encountering or that there was a problem at all…I just wanted to run faster. I diverted attention away from the negative feedback loop of flight and on to building a new fight response from running laps faster. This negative to positive change made such an amazing impact on my body that my conscious brain had to actually catch up with what I was now able to do subconsciously. If your brain remains positive, or happy, it will send more signals and release hormones so that the rest of the body will start to believe it. The brain loves novelty, and this was, indeed, a novel approach to "resetting" me in order to achieve what my subconscious once thought was impossible. Unknowingly, Leo had turned into a gym mouse, and this mouse had begun to fly.

"Comparing you to a mouse is quite humorous," a friend of mine later told me. "Scott, you must be Mighty Mouse."

The brain is an organ that serves as the center of our nervous system. Physiologically, the function of the brain is to exert centralized control over the other organs of the body. The brain acts on the rest of the body both by generating patterns of muscle activity (known as muscle maps) and by driving the secretion of hormones. This centralized control allows rapid and coordinated responses to changes in the environment. Some basic types of responsiveness, such as reflexes, can be mediated by the spinal cord or peripheral ganglia, but sophisticated, purposeful control of behavior based on complex sensory input requires the information integrating capabilities of a centralized brain. Simply put, by having me run laps, Ruth was able to find and execute my "reset trigger" when my brain went into flight mode.

It was as if my brain was telling me, "Scott, yes you *can* and *will* do this!" I thought of this as a *master reset button*, where my brain was so overloaded or hyperstimulated from running that it would reset and forget there was ever a problem at all. After the lap was completed, I would then come back to the activity I'd had trouble accomplishing, and I'd hammer through…with success every time. The strange part of this theory was that it did not work on folks who didn't have CP. These folks would run the lap and, because of their brains being "hyperstimulated," they would respond with diminished capability after their lap. More studies are needed, but I believe it had something to do with how the brains of people with CP have adapted over time to repairing and overcoming our condition.

This trigger worked successfully for over three years. Then the "reset" novelty started to subside. I began to think of running laps as punishment for doing something wrong, and my performance no longer improved like before. However, I was now operating at a much higher athletic level overall. I often wonder if this was a fallback to the old "give me a lap" routine many coaches over-employ on their students as punishment. Was I having some sort of flashback to my elementary school days? Or perhaps the novelty was just wearing thin, and my mind was getting bored of this "reset" protocol (perhaps Mighty Mouse's cape needed to be washed). The theory of overusing a trigger needed more research.

The power of positive thinking is remarkable—even more remarkable and powerful for folks with cerebral palsy. A lot of kids with CP develop extremely low self-esteem early on, largely due to society not understanding or accepting us. If this esteem is not turned positive, we often become paralyzed with a fear of failure, and complacency takes over, as I stated earlier. We need novel triggers in the gym and outside of the gym. For people with CP, the triggers must run deep to pull us out of our own heads and allow us to succeed. To improve my CP, Ruth had to first tackle my brain and build a "new me" inside my own head.

THE CIRCULAR-SAW TRIGGER

Ruth and I spent a lot of time training together outside the gym as well, working on my transformation over the years. From personally crafted workouts on the hiking trails to everyday tasks, Ruth pushed my way of thinking way beyond my own understanding. I always loved doing practical workouts, as I would later call them, with Ruth, workouts that I performed out in the "real world" rather than in the gym, where we essentially simulated what I should be doing outside the gym. Inside and outside the gym, she would correct my posture or alignment while I performed the tasks she assigned to me. Tapping or poking at various muscles and realigning my posture was a constant, and she had a unique way of "persuading me" to do what I was doing not with my left but with my right arm and hand.

On one such occasion, we were building outdoor chairs at her home. We used power tools, such as a circular saw, to take apart sixteen pallets to use as lumber. Using power tools was not new to me. After all, growing up with a dad who built and constantly maintained our lake house required a lot of hands-on work with power tools. One of my tasks on this particular day was to use the circular saw to cut the pallet boards to a measured length. The old me would have modified the cutting process. I would've found a way to use the saw left-handed to cut along the lines I had marked on each board. However, Ruth would not allow it. She insisted that I use my right hand.

Extremely nervous and unsure of what the outcome would be, I carefully switched hands. I took a deep breath, then slowly let it out. I then grasped the saw with my right hand and found the trigger with relative ease. I held the pallet board steady with my left hand and cautiously squeezed the trigger.

Surprisingly, the saw came to life. My heart pounded in my chest as my head worked to comprehend this strange new muscle movement while calculating my next move. Trigger pulled, saw on, now I had to engage my right arm and my chest to press evenly forward down the thin line while my left hand kept the board steady. *Sounds simple*, I thought, as another part of my mind was freaking out a little over just this part of a miracle. Before I knew it, I was cutting along the line, straight and true, dead reckoning—a line that was actually much easier to see as I cut it with my right hand. As I finished and the saw was revving down, I turned and looked at Ruth with sheer amazement. I think I even had a smile on my face as I realized I had successfully cut my first of many boards to come right-handed! I had done a task right-handed that I had only dreamed of as a youngster watching my dad build our house out on Lake Austin. Positive thinking changed my actions, with a little encouragement from my trainer.

EAT, DRINK, AND BE MERRY

Conditioning as an athlete or bodybuilder—whether one is aiming to lose fat, build lean muscle mass, or just improve cardiovascular endurance—all starts with the right activities at the right time. Eighty-five percent of a successful, healthy athletic program starts with proper eating (diet) and a good, steady cardio endurance routine. If you don't control what you eat while still increasing your cardiovascular endurance (burn rate), the productivity of everything you do as an athlete will be less than optimal. As part of building muscle and shredding fat, Ruth and I soon began to tackle how, when, and what I ate, along with increasing my cardiovascular endurance.

Ruth's early dedication to my transformation was simply amazing. I had never met anyone who cared for my health and physical growth in such a positive, caring manner as Ruth did. She went well beyond the boundaries of where any trainer I had ever known, or known of, would ever go. The belief she had in me and my abilities was way beyond my understanding or comprehension. I only knew that the more she poured into this project (me), the more

I wanted to show her and others I was not going to fail. I was not going to let her down. I wanted to show my trainer I was indeed worthy of her efforts and much, much more.

Modifying my diet, however, went beyond the training floor of her gym. She met me at the grocery store and showed me what "proper foods" I should be eating—and that included cutting the alcohol down to zero. She worked with me in designing a tailor-made weekly eating plan, complete with counting calories and weighing everything. I even had to purchase a digital scale and black plastic food containers that would hold my preplanned, premade meals for the week. I would log what I ate and when I ate in an app called MyFitness-Pal,[35] just released that same year. Everything was so clinical and structured, a concept far from what I was used to. We tracked my calories in (eats) and calories out (exercise). We tracked my workout progress, on the floor and off the floor, from a clinical, athletic training perspective. We would work out in her parking lot on all sorts of drills, including fast-twitch routines and other advanced cardiovascular concepts. We worked outside on hiking trails, in parking lots, and even at her house.

Mighty Mouse was now working Ruth's maze in record time.

"Make sure you drink plenty of water," Ruth would often remind me. As it turns out, there's a really good reason for ensuring that we remain hydrated during and after a workout. Hydration is one of the basics to doing a transformation right. Water not only helps us maintain proper electrolyte balance but is also critical for our kidneys to be able to flush out of our system all the waste by-products that accumulate during a workout, like proteins and enzymes from our muscle microtear breakdown and rebuilding process.

Drinking water, independent of other variables, can also increase metabolism, something I hadn't given much thought before my transformation began. By the time we feel thirsty, we are already dehydrated and in need of rehydration. Add to that an active workout and, if you are not drinking water, you are headed for real trouble. In my case, my kidneys started to hurt when I did not drink enough water. The resulting pain resembled back pain, but in reality, it was really my kidneys trying to flush out toxins without enough water in my system to do it properly. When I increased my water intake, my kidneys stopped hurting and my "back pain" went away.

Water is the best for rehydration. I learned to avoid sugary sports drinks due to the high caloric nature that tends to have a detrimental effect on weight loss / calorie burn. Just cold water for me, for those early thirty-minute or hour-long workouts with Ruth. I later had to step it up a notch by adding simple electrolytes to my water, to help with those workouts that were two hours or longer.

I felt as if I was in training for some sort of elite athletic competition. It was awesome, and I loved every moment of it. I had someone who believed in me, pushing me to excel in new ways not fully known to me. These were indeed exciting times.

COMPLIMENTS TO THE TIMID AND SCARED

About four months into my training with Ruth, I remember one day feeling like I was cowering behind her as she led me farther back into the gym than I had ever dared to venture before. We went back into the depths of this workout cave where all the dumbbells and free weights were located and all the serious, well-built muscle people lived. *This is the place where real weight lifters master their craft*, I thought. *I don't belong here.* We walked toward a bench, where Ruth began to teach me the basics of a dumbbell biceps curl and other free-weight moves that would later become second nature to me. I remember needing to use a wrist strap on my right hand to properly lift a mere five-pound dumbbell during that first session. A very large weight lifter commented to Ruth that it was "not right" for me to use a strap on that size weight. Ruth then told me to take a lap, not because I had trouble, but because she needed to "reeducate this guy."

I made two laps due to the length of her intense conversation with this self-proclaimed know-it-all. When I returned, he said to me that I was doing great, or something to that effect, then quickly gathered his stuff and left the gym. I later found out that Ruth had talked to him about me having cerebral palsy and that she was teaching proper functional weight lifting techniques and movements. This fellow was way too quick to judge, and it got him into serious trouble that day. I was already self-conscious about being in this part of the gym with "real weight lifters." Ruth was building my self-confidence and self-esteem along with my abilities, and she would not let anyone take this win from us. Ruth made me feel like a rock star at whatever I did, and I wanted to show her I could do more. I was turning into a real fighter on the workout floor.

One concept I had real trouble with during those early years, however, was accepting compliments. Trainers and other people started noticing what I was accomplishing and giving serious kudos on my performance and hard work, but I shrugged off their compliments. Ruth had to pull me aside one day. "These people are giving you genuine compliments, and you are not accepting them or acknowledging them well," she said. Deep down, I thought of their compliments as patronizing, like the ones from my days at the Austin CP Center or as a young "special" kid. It still felt like people might be complimenting me for something that was "easy." I didn't yet realize that I had become a true athlete, worthy of a compliment or two from the experts who knew what hard work really looked like. Accepting compliments would become a new task to add to my workouts. I had to start believing in myself the way these people who were giving me compliments did.

FAST-FORWARD ROW

Fast-forward a few years to 2018. February 1, to be exact. In a most unusual way, Ruth challenged me, along with others, to a Concept2 Nordic rowing competition at her gym. Speed and weight were not the object here, just cardio, stamina, and endurance over time. On that day, all the gyms in the region were in competition for the most time rowed by members. But Ruth's lack of communication upset me. I had traveled an hour to her gym for a one-on-one training session—a session I had really looked forward to. But upon arrival, Ruth said we were not going to train due to this special event. She had not texted or called to cancel our session. I was there, dressed to work out and ready for training. Peeved at this unexpected turn of events, I thought about walking out, but the *new* part of me wanted to show off and make her proud of how far I had come.

The Nordic rowing machine simulates a sculling type of rowing, like what I had observed on Lady Bird Lake (a.k.a. Town Lake) in downtown Austin over the years. Five or six people would sit in a long, thin boat, stroking in unison as the boat glided down the lake. These machines in the gym were simulator trainers for such a move. In this case, all rowing machines were preset at a medium to high level, and all we had to do was put our feet in the stirrups and row. I started around 4:30 p.m. that day, with a well-built guy to my left. There were two machines set side by side, and as we started out and hit our strides together, Ruth reminded me about proper alignment and movement consisting of full leg extensions and arm pulls at the end, with proper follow-through and recovery, breathing in on the return while extending my arms back out and bringing my knees back to my chest. Once I remembered the proper sequence and breathing pattern, I was all set.

We all encouraged each other to row just a little longer to bank more time for our gym, but about fifteen to twenty minutes into my run, the weight lifter to my left tuckered out and quit. I was surprised. After all, he was really built and looked like he could outrun me for sure. The next person to take over his slot on the other machine was a woman who looked to be in tip-top shape. She started out and matched my cadence. Again, I was stunned when after twenty minutes, she was done. With this, I got my second wind and decided to go for the gold. As others entered and left the race, I grew more emboldened to continue with every stroke. The crowd started to gather as time went on, cheering me on. Onlookers kept looking at my total time and the power of each stroke. The official recordkeeper even started paying extra attention as I racked up the distance and time.

Close to an hour and thirty minutes into the race, Ruth left the building for the evening without even a goodbye. I was not going to let this deflate me: I kept rowing. In fact, I kept rowing for a grand total of two hours and fifteen minutes. I rowed at a healthy, consistent pace, at the preset resistance level, for a total of twenty-seven thousand meters (16.8 miles). By the time I finished, I had trouble walking and standing, but I'd made it well beyond what I thought I could ever do. I'd made it longer than any other rower had done in this competition. My right grip had held firm, better than I expected, and my right leg kept pace with my left. My back, lats, and core were able to keep me stabilized, and my cardio endurance was in excellent shape. I had come a long way from that timid, scared, thin guy back by the free weights of my past. Unlike the other folks in that competition, I had successfully built a total-body makeover. Ruth told me that most people who only lift weights don't work on endurance. That's why I was able to outlast them all. She had known I could finish the race with no problem. I ended up burning 1,730 calories that evening, and for the next two weeks, I was the talk of the town in that gym.

DON'T FORGET TO BREATHE

Proper breathing techniques are also incredibly important while doing any physical fitness activity, such as cardio or weight lifting. Although most people think controlled breathing is only for cardio, proper breathing also affects how proficiently we lift weights. The branch of the autonomic nervous system that manages our body's internal processes is broken into two parts: the sympathetic nervous system, which is responsible for our "fight or flight" response and controls our state of readiness, and the parasympathetic nervous system, responsible for the "rest and digest" state, which controls our ability to rest and the recovery of our reproductive system. Both of these branches of our nervous system are influenced by how and when we breathe.

When weight lifters lift weights, we are primarily using our sympathetic nervous system in fight mode, as mentioned earlier. While in fight mode, we need to be able to control breathing to maintain focus, to keep oxygen flowing to muscles, and to decrease recovery time between reps, which also slows down heart rate. Unfortunately, most novice weight lifters don't acquire this basic knowledge or training on how to breathe correctly. Even though I was an experienced scuba diver who had been taught how to breathe while diving, weight lifting and athletics that build endurance require a whole different breathing technique. Breathing conservation is the key in scuba diving. This is not so in weight lifting or cardio training.

At its basic level, the weight lifter must inhale deeply on the beginning of the muscle movement and exhale on the muscle contraction, or when moving against gravity—never holding the breath. This allows the blood and the brain to receive sufficient oxygen during exercise. Deep breathing from the diaphragm, known as diaphragmatic breathing, helps oxygen reach the lowest regions of the lungs, where there's more blood and a greater exchange of oxygen and carbon dioxide.[36]

People do this naturally when there is no clear and present danger, but when weight lifting or in fight-or-flight mode, we tend to shallow breathe or hold our breath altogether and must consciously think about deep breathing until this practice is ingrained into our muscle memory. Without exception, we are to always aim for diaphragmatic breathing when working out.

As it turns out, coaches and many trainers have it all wrong. We are not supposed to breathe in through our nose and out through the mouth. Why is this? As Garrett Salpeter explains in his book *The NeuFit Method*,

> When people exhale through their nose, they preserve more of that carbon dioxide–rich air in the upper throat and chest so they can take it in on the next inhale. Exhaling through the nose increases the amount of carbon dioxide in the body, which supports healthy blood flow and oxygen delivery, as well as balancing blood sugar and stabilizing the nervous system.[37]

Boy, did I have this concept wrong when I first started training! Almost every time, I would breathe incorrectly or forget to breathe altogether. Holding one's breath seems to be very common in novice weight lifters who have not been properly trained. I had to learn how to intentionally slow down my breathing and reduce the volume of air exchange to train my brain and nervous system to stay relaxed—even when my body was hungry for air—and teach my body to tolerate higher carbon dioxide levels while breathing in sufficient oxygen for my muscles. It took a long time to master breathing and keeping count of my reps all at the same time. It reminded me of patting my head while rubbing my stomach, which I still have not mastered. When I do breathe correctly, I actually notice a big difference in how much I am able to lift and how long I am able to stay in the game while my rep count goes up. During endurance workouts like cardio, these techniques also helped me run farther for longer periods of time.[38]

HIGH-ALTITUDE TRAINING

Back when I was first learning to swim, as a baby, Kelly Osness was there at what seemed to be endless summer water-ski tournaments. Kelly ended up drafted as my de facto "babysitter." We fast became best buds over those many years. In fact, from the very first time I was held outside my immediate family, Kelly was there holding me as an infant, with such a unique, kind, and caring spirit. Many years later, in early April of 2012, I decided to visit Kelly and her husband, Chris Osness, at their mountainside home in Gunnison, Colorado. This was during the time when the seeds had been planted but before my transformation had officially taken root; needless to say, it was a very low point in my life. You could say it was during my "baseline" period—that point in time I had come to understand as the beginning of my transformation journey.

A year into my transformation, in 2013, I had a desire to go back and visit Chris and Kelly. Ruth King and I talked at length about my return to Gunnison for a respite "getaway" vacation. It would be an escape from the grind and hustle of city life where I could also mix things up a bit with my training. I wanted to return to Gunnison to visit old friends once again and flex my newly acquired muscles and cardiovascular system. I also wanted to stretch my legs on nearby mountains and have some high-altitude adventures. Ruth thought it was a great idea.

Upon my return to Gunnison, Kelly and Chris treated me to their hometown hospitality once again. They outfitted me with the latest gear from their store, Treads 'N' Threads,[39] for my upcoming Gunnison adventures and introduced me to their good friend Jane.

Jane Tunnadine was the owner and operator of Colorado Fitness, a fantastic little gym located just south of Main off Tomichi Avenue and Fourteenth Street.

Upon learning of my transformation story, passion, and progression, Jane welcomed me as she would an old friend and offered her place as my Gunnison "base camp" for whenever I wished to visit. My Austin friends could not quite understand why I would go up to the mountains and work out in a gym and not just outside. Resistance and cardio training takes many forms, I asserted. As a "Texas boy," working out at Jane's gym would provide a controlled environment for my body to adjust to the Gunnison altitude and thinner air, a place to prepare for those treks up on the mountain.

It did not take long. Before I knew it, I was performing at a higher level and lasting longer on my daily workouts. Something about the atmosphere energized me. Perhaps it was the cold, crisp air or the psychological impact of looking out at mountains in the distance while working out. Whatever the case, it really motivated me. My body took to the environment as if I were a native, and I wanted to soak it all up.

I would routinely perform resistance and cardio endurance workouts at Colorado Fitness in the mornings and then meet Kelly and Chris at their shop, just down the street, for a bite to eat on Main Street, at either the W Cafe or the Gunnisack Cowboy Bistro Restaurant and Bar. Then I'd hike up at Hartman Rocks or out at Mill Creek in the afternoons. At first, it was tough for me to make it through without lengthy rest breaks, but as time progressed and my body adjusted, I really got into the game and pushed harder by the hill. My body loved the novelty of these static and dynamic training programs.

HARTMAN ROCKS

One of my favorite spots that Kelly and Chris introduced me to was Hartman Rocks Recreation Area. Hartman Rocks is located five minutes south of the Gunnison–Crested Butte Regional Airport, or about fifteen bike minutes southwest of downtown Gunnison.

While on my first mountain hike at Hartman with Kelly and Chris back in 2012, we stopped to rest and have a snack at an outcrop of rocks that provided a great view of Gunnison to the north. Kelly snapped a photo of me eating a snack on a spot overlooking Gunnison in the background and jokingly dubbed it "Scott's Spot." Unbeknownst to us at that time, this photo would later become a very special memento and serve as my *baseline transformation picture*, which would be the catalyst for everything to come.

MILL CREEK HIKES

On my 2013 visit, when I was not hiking with Kelly or working out at Colorado Fitness, I would often travel just a few miles up Ohio Creek Road (CR 730) from Chris and Kelly's home to Mill Creek, where Mill Creek Road (CR 727) ends, to hike the trails off in their "backyard." Mill Creek sits at an elevation of 9,500 feet and offers some simply majestic hiking.

I would take my hiking boots and poles, GPS, water, and a snack or two and head up there for the entire afternoon, exploring trail after trail, adventuring farther and farther in, higher up, farther back than the hike before—always gazing at nature and all the wonders that were about. I was out in the "wild," and I'd forget that I was training or doing cardio. These hikes became my "fun workouts."

THE CASTLES

I also hiked the Castles. Starting at 8,900 feet, I would gain close to 4,900 feet in elevation as I ascended to 12,496 feet. Not bad for a cardiovascular climb, and not an easy one. The hike up the Mill Castle Trail to Storm Pass and back is about fifteen and a half miles and is one of the most scenic hikes I have experienced in Colorado.

The hike back down tended to be easier for me, but the miles and elevation descent often took a toll on my legs. I was grateful for my hiking poles on each descent down the mountain trail.

All of this in Gunnison's backyard. I simply loved working out on these mountains! This is why we train inside a gym: to be able to go higher and farther out in the wild.

BURNING THE MIDNIGHT OIL

Back at home, prebreakfast carb-depleted cardio sessions had been a favorite homework assignment of Ruth's as well. This was meant to hyperstimulate my metabolism by burning fat (called ketosis) instead of digested carbohydrates (say, from eating breakfast). The basic premise of this workout was that within thirty minutes of waking up early in the morning, I would hit cardio for forty-five minutes at a consistent pace of 65 to 75 percent max heart rate, then eat a healthy breakfast no more than fifteen minutes after cardio. In those early days of my transformation, Ruth had me wake up, hurry down to her gym, and do this early morning torture session. Most of my close friends know that

I am not a morning person; waking up early is not something I like to do in the first place. Putting cardio on top of rushing down to the gym within thirty minutes on an empty stomach tends to be challenging in itself. My old way of thinking told me that not having morning coffee or anything but water was just plain wrong, and my body did not react well to this forced labor at first. Just walking without stimulants was hard enough.

However, novel approaches do work, and I was up for the challenge! My first prebreakfast carb-depleted cardio session was difficult. I think I ended up taking a two-hour nap right after eating. As time progressed, these sessions became easier as my body adapted to the routine, and I started burning fat faster than I had ever been able to before. After a while, I ended up doing a prebreakfast carb-depleted cardio workout, eating two small meals spaced two hours apart, then heading back to the gym to lift weights (resistance training), followed by another high-protein meal.

Ruth then introduced me to nutrition in the form of vitamins and supplements, along with the correct fluids to drink. I even started taking pre-workout and post-workout products such as N.O.-XPLODE or Cellucor C4 and protein mixes. Now I really began to shred and lean out with astounding results.

By the end of year one of my transformation, on August 23, 2013, Ruth asked me to take a new photo of myself in the exact same pose at the same spot I had visited in 2012 while hiking Hartman Rocks in Gunnison—Scott's Spot. She asked me to send her the photo as soon after as possible. Not giving it much thought, I took another photo as requested and sent it to her via text while still up on the mountain. In real time, she cropped in the "baseline" photo of me next to this new photo, and bam! The comparison she sent back to me while still up on that mountain was simply astounding.

It was all the proof I needed. My transformation had officially begun. My new photo, along with the measurements she had not told me of until that moment, was amazing!

I now weighed in at 163 pounds and 13 percent body fat, and it showed in that photo. That was a decrease of 35 pounds and 26 percent body fat reduction in one year's time! Kelly pointed out that it had taken a while for me to make it up that mountain at Hartman Rocks a year prior (2012) and that I had needed several lengthy rest breaks for recovery along the trek. But on the second climb up that same mountain, in 2013, I actually had to wait for Kelly and Chris, and they lived at this elevation—that's a 180-degree change in my stamina, cardiovascular fitness, and physique in just one year! My hard work, Jane's gym, and Ruth's Austin-based personal training was starting to pay dividends. This was to be the start of an eight-year transformation project.

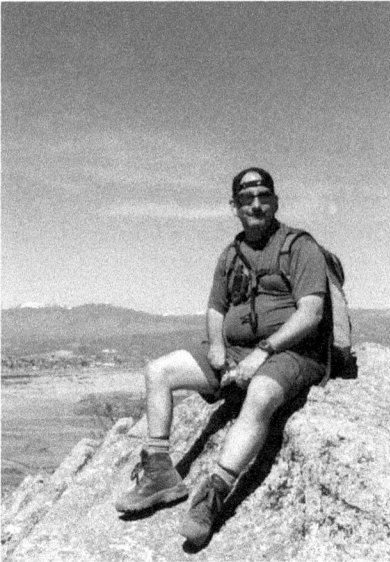

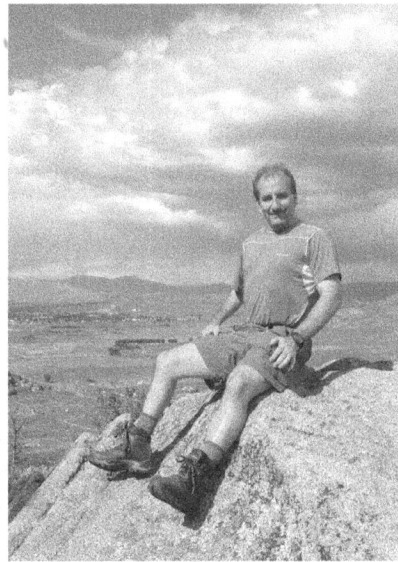

Scott before transformation (2012) and after one year of transformation training (2013), Hartman Rocks

Mighty Mouse needed a new set of tights.

TRAIN OR DIE—SURVIVAL OF THE FITTEST

When Ruth was promoted into a management position and unable or unwilling to train clients anymore, I had the opportunity to meet and train with Brian Williams beginning in October of 2015. Ruth paired me with Brian at her new club up in the Round Rock area because she trusted that Brian would continue the growth and effective, safe practices that I required. We quickly developed a bond, continued to break barriers together, and reached heights that Brian said I was so willing to pursue because of my "raw determination and unbreakable spirit." Brian went on to say, "Every goal we accomplished, every hurdle we jumped, and every wall we broke through—until we had to start creating new objectives to achieve—it was fun to work with Scott."

Sports and exercise had been a part of Brian's life for as long as he could remember. He considered himself a natural athlete, and because of that, he was able to excel in many different athletic arenas. However, it wasn't until he lost his father in a tragic car accident in 1997 that Brian turned in the direction of physical therapy. Brian's father had suffered the paralyzing effects of polio early in life. Although he had survived polio, he had diminished use of one of his legs. Brian had always thought that if only his father had received physical therapy to correct the neuromuscular imbalance caused by polio, he may not have been in that accident that took his life. Because of this, he wanted to pursue the career path of physical therapy, where he could help others be healthier, be stronger, and live longer. This is when he began the journey to finish his degree in kinesiology (exercise sports science) at Texas State University and ultimately complete his bachelor's in kinesiology, with honors, in 2003.

While finishing his degree, he started personal training. He received his first personal training certification with the International Sports Sciences Association (ISSA) and began training independently in the Greater Austin area. Although his initial intention was to coach and to teach physical therapy, he fell in love with the freedom of being his own boss, the gratification of changing lives as a trainer, and the great relationships he fostered. Once he completed his education, he found it difficult to compete with the world of independent training, so he joined the Gold's Gym team in 2004. Fourteen years later, he had acquired several more certifications through NESTA, NCCPT, NCSF, FiTOUR (Boot Camp, Aqua Fitness, and Group), and SPIN (Ride).

Brian knows that everyone's situation is different and that if you take the time to really listen and communicate, you can always figure out a way to make a tangible difference in someone's life.

Back then, Brian and I trained at a Gold's Gym that paralleled a penal-colony workout yard you might see in the movies. There were lots of characters and tough-looking "inmates" around. I first felt a little intimidated by my lack of body build compared to these fellas but soon realized that I could actually hang in this place. Brian did amazing things with me back then, and I was stoked with our work.

One day while in session with Brian, I was approached by several well-built fellas. We exchanged fist bumps, and they said they were quite moved by my workout spirit, intense determination, and drive. I was taken aback by the respect and camaraderie they showed me. It was a brand-new peer-exchange experience that I had not been exposed to in any sort of workout or physical capacity before.

One particularly large bodybuilder asked me for my shirt size. Perplexed at such a question, I answered as firmly as I could muster. He then turned and walked off without a word. A few minutes later, he returned and gave me a long-sleeved, black hoodie with a skull and barbells on the front that read "Train or Die" and "Survival of the Fittest" in bold letters on the back. He told me upon presenting it that he made these for dudes who had high training standards and who he knew would go far. He only gave them to worthy bodybuilders, he said, at no charge. I still cherish the hoodie and wear it to my winter workout sessions to this day.

HARTMAN ROCKS WALL OF FAME

For a total of seven years, I returned to that same spot on Hartman Rocks to capture progression photos, along with measurements of my transformation journey:

1. April 13, 2012—198 pounds, 39 percent body fat (baseline)

2. August 23, 2013—163 pounds, 13 percent body fat

3. October 20, 2014—163 pounds, 11 percent body fat

4. July 13, 2015—164 pounds, 10 percent body fat

5. July 19, 2016—152 pounds, 8 percent body fat

6. September 15, 2017—151 pounds, 11 percent body fat

7. October 9, 2018—160 pounds, 13 percent body fat, with an added bonus: a well-defined six-pack

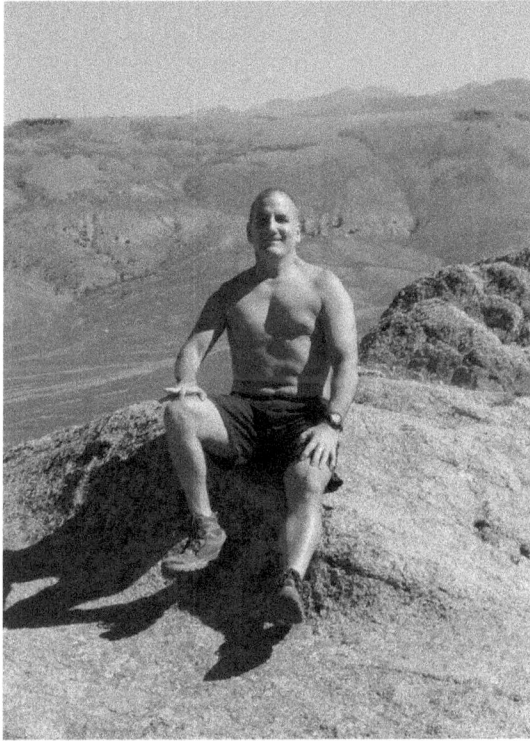

October 2018 transformation picture

I had a well-defined six-pack by year seven (September 2018). My doctors up to this point told me I could never achieve a four-pack, much less a six-pack, due to my CP—but I'm getting ahead of myself again.[40] To say my transformation was going like gangbusters was an understatement. I was so stoked, and I think both Ruth and Brian were so proud of their work with me.

PART 6

Deepening Faith

Making All Things New

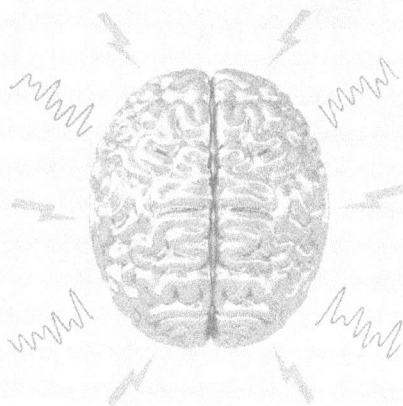

Finding Faith on the Workout Floor

"I know how to live humbly, and I know how to abound. I am accustomed to any and every situation—to being filled and being hungry, to having plenty and having need. I can do all things through Christ, who gives me strength. Nevertheless, you have done well to share in my affliction..."

—PHILIPPIANS 4:12–14

THIS IS AN INCREDIBLE, SPECIAL PASSAGE THAT IS NEAR AND DEAR TO my heart. These words were placed in my heart early in my transformation. I had needed inspiration during my workouts to stay motivated and focused through the darkest hours of my training, and there were many, many dark times.

Verse 13 in particular, "I can do all things through Christ, who gives me strength," was just what was needed. In those early days of training, it had been hard to remain faithful on that workout floor. I had been frustrated and losing hope. I wondered why my body was not doing what my trainer knew it could do. I did not understand why my body wouldn't do what I told it to.

197

Today, I recite this verse before my workouts and repeat it often on the days when all seems lost and futile or when I am not sure I can achieve more reps or more laps. Even now, before every workout, I recite this verse to keep myself focused and humble on the workout floor so that I will remember this:

I am His vessel, for His purposes, for His glory.

I also listen to a preset playlist of music when I work out on my own. The music helps my body perform better and stay focused. By engaging different parts of my brain to work in concert, I tend to do better (more on this topic to come).

I first noticed the concept of engaging different parts of the brain when training for my first 5K run up in Gunnison, Colorado. I would train for this run on a treadmill at a five-mile-per-hour pace to the same soundtrack, over and over for five kilometers, then ten kilometers, at sea level in Austin, Texas. When the day came and I was up in Gunnison, out on that mountain trail, I kicked the music up, and there I was once again, in the zone. I had unknowingly conditioned my brain to run to the soundtrack and focus on things other than all my pain. My brain knew just what to do. The music helped engage my motor centers to work in concert with the auditory centers of my brain. I finished the 2013 Gunnison 5K Color Run in fourth place, at 7,703 feet above sea level.

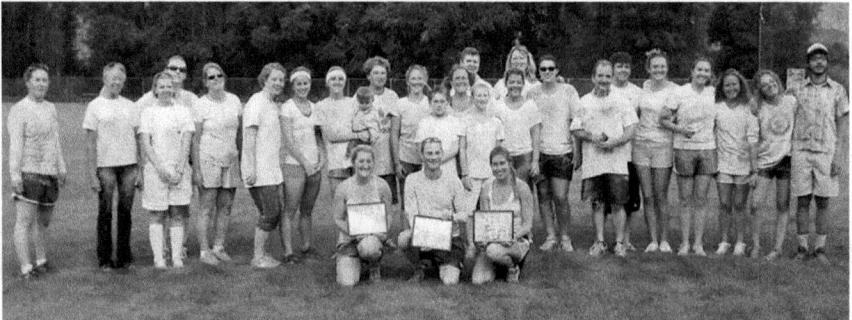

Scott's first 5K Color Run in Gunnison, Colorado, finishing in fourth place

Faith has been a strong proponent of my life ever since 2001. Knowing that I am a child of God who has been created to perform certain tasks and teach others to achieve things that are way beyond their own understanding has been a great joy to live out. Having cerebral palsy has taught me that it is not by my will, but by His will, that I can do all things and help pave the road for others by pioneering new, innovative approaches and PT techniques to help others along their journey. With every workout, every milestone, and every triumph, I just smile and think, *Wow, that's cool, God. Show me more and lead others like You have led me.*

RESETTING THE BAR

I had started to show great advancements on and off the workout floor by 2014. I began to get the notion that perhaps I actually *was* a real athlete. Up to this point, deep inside, I had been thinking of PT in the sense of physical therapy, not personal training, as is applied to a *real* athlete. Again, it was that childhood thought pattern, so ingrained in me, that failure was just around the corner at every turn. By this time (before Ruth went into management the next year), Ruth was going way beyond what a normal trainer would do in helping me achieve great gains.

By year three (2014), with effort, I was able to start my car right-handed. A huge first for me! Simple, right? But try this after only using your left hand for thirty-plus years because you don't have enough dexterity in your right hand to twist that little metal key. Then start "attempting" to use your less-dominant right hand with CP. Muscle memory had to be changed. This was a real turning point for me. What else could—and would—I ultimately be able to do right-handed?

Functional lifting, using common items like tires and even rocks out on the trail, soon became part of my workout routine. It was fun having a real champion behind me, motivating me forward, and I really wanted to please my trainer—someone who really believed in me.

I began to wonder where the bar for my abilities actually was. How high could I go?

Remember the transformation pictures I took in "Scott's Spot" in Gunnison? Every year, I would go back to Gunnison, to that same exact spot, to take a new progression photograph to compare to my baseline of April 2012. And every year, I would see a new, leaner, more defined, more muscular me in the photos. I started to look really *built*, and that's when I had the epiphany that I was indeed an athlete and bodybuilder. Mighty Mouse was now confident in his abilities and wanted to fly.

Gold's national headquarters showed my transformation picture from my first year, along with my bio, to all their trainers in a meeting about transforming clients in 2013. By 2014, I began to win my local gym's transformation challenge for my age bracket, and this was a real game changer for me—to be listed on their Wall of Fame (at several Gold's Gym locations). I won three local Gold's challenges for my age bracket over the years. I was featured in the lifestyle section of my local newspaper, the *Austin American-Statesman*,[41] and had my background and story featured in a couple of PhD papers.[42] I started to think that I was on to something, and I wanted to share it with others. Others who had given up, who had been taught that "No" was to be their standard response. That they would not be able to do more. I was becoming a trailblazer to lead others like me.

By 2015, I began to actively raise the bar, to shoot for what I could not have imagined just a few years prior. New personal records with Ruth occurred faster and faster. First, I successfully performed an unassisted bench press (forty-five-pound Olympic bar, plus ten pounds) on August 5, 2015, something I had thought I would never be able to do with CP. When Ruth showed me that I could gain the strength and dexterity to do it, I was all in.

- January 26, 2018: I caught a lacrosse ball right-handed for the first time.

- Just a few months later, on June 1, 2018, I maxed out a T-bar row with four plates (180 pounds).

- June 7, 2018: I performed a dead lift lockout of 315 pounds (six plates).

- November 19, 2018: I was now bench-pressing a 45-pound plate (per side) for a total of 135 pounds…a huge milestone from not being able to do a bench press unassisted, *ever*, just a short time before.

As a result of all my new muscle growth happening so fast, Ruth would often perform myofascial release, a method of eliminating and easing trigger points and restoring tissue integrity and normal functioning. She would usually do this with her hands. We started in those early days by working on my right arm with my mom's old wooden rolling pin. Then Ruth worked up to using a hard foam roller or small hard rubber ball, before or during most of my workouts. Then she graduated to a small white PVC pipe or red stick that she would use all over my body while I lay on the workout floor, screaming in agony almost every time. This became a Pavlovian "dreaded" technique for me that involved applying extraordinarily strong pressure to the tissues that surround, support, and connect my muscles. In most cases, the pain was temporary. For me, an extreme amount of pain was part of my daily training.

During one such session, I was lying on my stomach on the workout floor, screaming like a wounded wildebeest, when I felt a pop and the pain subsided. She had somehow "sadistically" reached up behind my right shoulder blade and "unlocked" my frozen right scapula. Manually, she got my subscapular muscle to fully retract, and then she taught me how to fully retract my shoulder blade on my own, to achieve equal mobility in both shoulders, allowing me to "push" the Olympic bar higher, farther, and stronger than ever before! This was significant because, up to this point, my doctors and medical staff had told me that obtaining a six-pack would be impossible because the subscapular muscle on my right side was locked and unable to fully retract, which prevented such gains.

By February 16, 2018, I achieved full right shoulder mobility and scapula retraction without my triceps overcompensating, and by September of that year, I had a fully developed six-pack. This was the year that I was professionally tanned and photographed with a full, well-defined six-pack at 160 pounds (13 percent body fat) for that year's Gold's transformation photo. My doctors were dumbfounded.

As I stated in the introduction, that's when I decided to start writing this book. If I could do so much in such a short time span, what could others achieve with proper motivation? I wanted to share the story of my triumph over cerebral palsy and lead others to even greater triumphs in their own lives. I doubt author Robert Kraus ever dreamed that, as a little boy, I would choose his book to read about a little lion, subconsciously relating my life to Leo's. Leo may have been a late bloomer, but he would become a great leader of lions in the days to come. As Mighty Mouse, I outran every maze they put me in, and I learned how to fly higher than any bar they said I could not reach.

IS THERE EVEN A BAR?

Where was the bar for what I could actually achieve? Was there even a bar anymore? I had come to understand that the bar of success is an artificial limit imposed on us by others or inside our own heads, and I desperately wanted to teach others that they, too, could move their bars up, up, and away. Mighty Mouse had learned to fly, and so could you!

STRETCH LIKE NEVER BEFORE

Over the years, I have found that prayer and hope are enormously powerful tools in the treatment of CP. With these tools, as an adult, I was blessed with my first team of highly competent professionals to help me in this next phase of my transformation. For so many years, I had been told over and over that there was *nothing* I could do regarding the movement of my arm and rotation of my hand. My arm, they said, must have formed some restriction, like calcium buildup, and I would never be able to straighten it, *ever*! And as for my hand rotation, they said it was too late to do anything about it.

"Scott has had CP all his life, and there is little chance he will ever get better," the doctors had said.

As a reminder, from an early age, I looked different from other kids. I was not "normal." I was a small, skinny kid with cerebral palsy, and as a survival mechanism, I developed into a shy, timid little boy. My CP affects the entire right side of my body, and as I grew, my right arm and right leg were underdeveloped.

I was unable to fully straighten my right arm like normal kids did. With spasticity in full rigor at various times of the day, my arm loved to curl up (known as *centralization*) to my chest, and my right hand would bend down and in. As I used my left arm and hand more, my right would just retreat to my chest, and this became a visual strain on my psyche. Over the early years, I would passively attempt to utilize my right arm more, but the techniques I employed would not last or would fail outright, and any forward progress was halted. My right-side calf muscle was also noticeably smaller, and if I did not place equal weight onto my right side, the spasticity in my right leg would compel my right heel to raise off the floor, causing my right knee to bend and hips to go out of alignment.

My altered gait also was distinct, with a right-side limp. As part of a competition water-skiing family, not being able to effectively use my arms or legs meant that I would never build a water-skiing résumé. This weighed heavily on such a little boy's psyche, for water-skiing was everything to my dad—and as hard as I would try, failure was always close at hand. My leg was easy to hide, but my arm…my arm was a telltale sign that skinny Scott had something wrong with him. I picked up on the cues from everyone around me, especially other kids who had not yet learned the social etiquette of refraining from drawing attention to such "deformities." Kids don't hide emotions very well, and I felt all of that, all the time.

* * *

Dr. Karen Pape expressed the following in her book, *The Boy Who Could Run but Not Walk*:

> Much of spasticity is a habit of the brain and body. It begins when the brain is damaged, and the body tries to move against gravity. The nerves send a signal to the muscles that are easiest to activate—the flexor muscles of the upper body and the extensor muscles of the lower body. These muscles inhibit the muscles that are supposed to be their partners in creating a fluid movement, and in doing so they destroy the elegant dance that most of us take for granted. Every time the child tries to move a hand or stand up, the bully muscles get stronger and the partner muscles get weaker. Eventually, after thousands of repetitions, it forms a facilitated network in the brain that guides this awkward movement.

Dr. Pape calls this "a negative feedback loop" that "springs into action every time the person wants to move."[43]

Early in my work with Ruth, we worked on stretching my right hand and arm—or, more accurately, improving my grip, arm extension, and hand rotation. She suggested that we investigate outpatient physical therapy to determine full range of motion, ability to stretch the muscles and tendons that restricted the full extension of my arm, and full rotation of my right hand from pronation (palms down) through neutral (thumbs up, like Fonzie) to palms-up supination ("Please, sir, may I have some more, please?"). Ruth had a working theory but still required more data to prove it. Full right-hand supination had never been possible up to this point, but she was sure that I could obtain this "impossibility," contrary to what my doctors had told me all my life. I was referred to St. David's Outpatient Rehabilitation in Austin, Texas, for evaluation and to determine a suitable treatment plan in October 2015. After an initial visit and evaluation, the therapists were certain that I *would* be able to extend my range of motion for both arm extension and hand rotation, but by how much was still in question.

I was stoked! I mean, really, *really* excited. Something I had been told was impossible was, in fact, not.

During our research and physical therapy plan, Ruth and I had sought assistance from St. David's for their evaluation, techniques, and information about splinting my right arm to achieve the "dynamic stretch" required to lengthen the tight tendons in my arm and hand. I soon began physical therapy at St. David's.

Measurements were taken, scans were performed, and the possibility for improvement became stronger with each session. My St. David's physical therapist soon offered hope and a valuable lead that would ultimately change my range of motion like no other past attempt had been able to achieve.

I soon received more good news. St. David's had set up a consultation with Matt Patocki, an occupational therapist from Dynasplint Systems. Dynasplint, which was founded in 1981, was originally named Therapeutic Appliances. The idea occurred to founder George R. Hepburn while working with a patient at Knollwood Manor nursing home. Two years later, a prototype was built and named the Universal Knee and Elbow Extension System.

The Universal Knee and Elbow Dynasplint was crafted to be used on the elbow or knee—one unit for both joints. While an elderly patient in a nursing home helped prove the Dynasplint concept, she unfortunately didn't live long enough to enjoy the full benefits that the product's use provided for her severely contracted knees. But her legacy as the first user confirmed the "dynamic stretch," as it was called, over time was a proven treatment mode.

Simply put, Dynasplint Systems are bilateral, spring-loaded tensioning devices that help to increase joint range of motion (ROM) in patients experiencing ROM deficits due to shortened connective tissue. Each splint is designed to gently stretch the affected joint at its end range. By applying a low-load stretch with its simple and adjustable tension, the Dynasplint slowly elongates the tight tissue, thereby providing the proper range of motion for extension. The low-load, prolonged-duration stretch technology delivers a biomechanically correct stimulus to create a permanent length change in shortened connective tissue (muscles, tendons, and ligaments).

What is more amazing is that these devices are available for infant, pediatric, and adult patients and are easy to use. They are fairly comfortable and usually worn at rest. Boy, I wish I had discovered this technology as a small kid!

Since the first use in 1981, Dynasplint has provided dynamic splints in various configurations across the entire world for helping restore lost range of motion in all of the peripheral body joints. They now supply over ninety different configurations of this simple yet sophisticated splinting system to the medical rehabilitation marketplace...and I was next in line for a go.

My case files were reviewed by Jon Hanczaryk, an insurance and contracting manager at Dynasplint. Jon and his team provided various white papers and treatment protocols, which provided promising results for people like me with spastic CP. My prior progress with manual manipulation of my right arm and right hand made me a perfect candidate for Dynasplint's Elbow Extension (E1800) and Supination/Pronation (E1802) devices.

I met with Dynasplint occupational therapy (OT) representatives along with my St. David's PT staff. I first started with the extension splint, at night only.

We added the right-hand rotation splint one month later. Known as the Supination/Pronation Dynasplint System, this device was a bit more complicated and reminded me of a halo system for grafting broken bones together or something from *Star Trek*'s Borg Collective. "Scott is Borg," my friends would soon joke while I was in this splint.

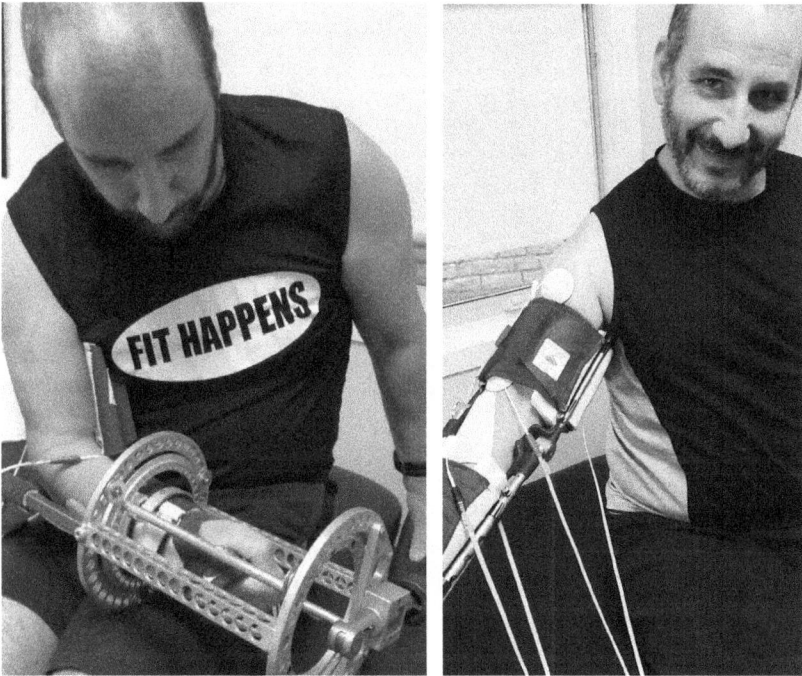

With Dynasplint's Elbow Extension (E1800) and Supination/Pronation (E1802) devices with Neubie ESTIM pads placed on arm to condition muscles

I loved all the technology that Dynasplint offered. I wanted to learn the theory behind these devices and witness the anticipated results for myself. I decided even back then that my long-term goal would be to share what I had learned and experienced with others who would come after me—others who needed help just like I did.

Mighty Mouse's brain was no longer in a locker. Results with both splints were quite promising, and over time, both were doing the trick. However, I quickly ran into a problem. My insurance carrier at that time would not cover the large cost of these devices and would only cover a small fraction of the OT at St. David's. In a letter from Aetna, I was told that there was "no established benefit that Dynasplinting or PT would bring any substantial change to the patient." They outright denied my claim. Even though Dynasplint produced white papers[44] and doctor-direct evidence,[45] including my own case study as proof, they still would not cover any of the treatment.

Our insurance system seemed to be against sufferers of CP due to a lack of understanding or willingness to admit they had no idea what they were talking about.

I was determined, if not more emboldened, to change this for all of us with CP! I had learned in business school, years back, that the fastest way to get someone's attention is to hit them where it counts. In this case, in the wallet. My first step was to fire my insurance provider and seek coverage with another company.

I started calling all the providers available to me at the time, and the representatives at Blue Cross and Blue Shield of Texas were eager to help. I presented my case and asked if they covered renting Dynasplints for treating spastic CP. Not only did they cover this treatment and believe it was beneficial for their clients, but they also asked if I would prefer to just buy the splints outright due to the long-term nature of my PT treatment plan. Needless to say, Aetna was dropped, with a stern letter to their medical advisory committee citing a lack of care for their policyholders with CP. I was relieved that Blue Cross was now my insurance carrier and they were very open to treating people with CP. As a side note, Jon Hanczaryk and his team of experts at Dynasplint worked alongside me every step of the way, and they were instrumental in helping pave the way both in treatment and in managing my insurance nightmare, which persisted for over two and a half years. Results don't lie. Dynasplint has allowed me to obtain full manual assisted extension and full supination within three years of use.

The next step was to activate my muscles to do autonomous movement without dynamic splint assistance. Simply put, I would need to learn to move my body using my brain and muscles (neuromuscular) without any help from splints. Up to this point, I had achieved pronation to supination through manual passive muscle manipulation, either by Dynasplint or manual PT range-of-motion techniques. I now had to learn to consciously activate my own muscles to achieve full rotation and extension of my right arm and hand by my own will. To accomplish this, I began the task of researching everything I could find on ESTIM and muscle stimulation technology.

I found two fascinating ESTIM stories during my research—one involving electric eels and the other involving actor Bruce Lee. It is interesting that electrical stimulation dates back to ancient times, when *electric eels* were used to treat spines and limbs to relieve pain and treat patents. The other fascinating story I uncovered was that the famous actor Bruce Lee actually employed a rudimentary high-voltage, alternating current form of ESTIM obtained from Japan, to stimulate his muscles during and between various workouts and on the set of his movies between takes. Some reports even suggest that this form of EMS ultimately destroyed the balance between Lee's nervous system and body and that it may have contributed to his death on July 20, 1973, at the age of thirty-two. (The most likely causes of his death were suggested to be mental issues, overwork, or overuse of high-voltage EMS.) According to a website about Lee's death, fellow actor Yuan Jie utilized this kind of machine from Japan and died of unknown causes as well, one year after Lee's death.[46]

Now, where to find me an eel to further my research?

A safe form of ESTIM was to be my next quantum leap forward in overall ability—a leap that would not be possible today if not for Dynasplint's PT/OT professionals and their medical systems, along with St. David's recommendation and work. As part of researching and writing this book, I have maintained a strong alliance with Dynasplint, providing my case study as further evidence that their splints, coupled with PT/OT, do provide positive benefits for people with CP.

PART 7

New Beginnings

*Sometimes You Must Step
Backwards to Move Forward*

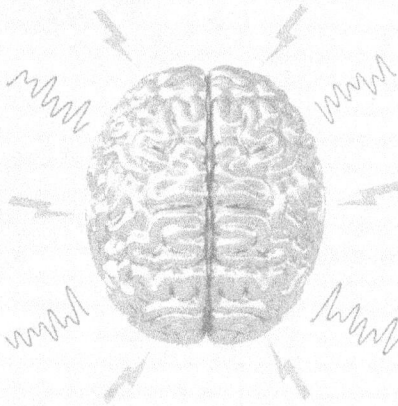

The Boy Who Could Run but Not Walk

In the book I mentioned earlier, *The Boy Who Could Run but Not Walk*, Dr. Karen Pape describes treating a premature infant named Daniel while at the Hospital for Sick Children (SickKids) in Toronto, Canada, in the 1970s.[47] Dr. Pape explains that Daniel was born at twenty-six weeks and weighed only 1.5 pounds. In his first week of life, he developed a major bleed in the right side of his brain, damaging the areas that would normally control the left side of his body. Daniel survived, but the common wisdom of doctors in those days was that the damage to his brain was irreversible and would lead to permanent disability with both gross and fine motor skills. Traditional therapy was initiated, and Dr. Pape started to track Daniel's progress as he grew. As a child, Daniel walked with a limp on his left side, landing on the front half of his left foot (a spastic toe-heel gait). He walked without a limp on his right side, with a regular heel-toe gait. His left arm hung at his side and did not swing normally when Daniel walked. His right side was unaffected, and his right arm functioned normally. Dr. Karen Pape diagnosed Daniel with left-sided hemiplegia cerebral palsy.

Several years had passed after his discharge from the neonatal follow-up clinic where Dr. Pape worked, since they only tracked kids up to three to four years post-birth. One day, Daniel's mother called Dr. Pape with news. Daniel was now playing soccer on a competitive able-bodied league. Dr. Pape thought to herself, *The hell he is*, but actually said to his mother, "Oh?" Dr. Pape didn't believe her. After all, Daniel being able to play competitive soccer was outside her—and most doctors'—understanding of hemiplegia. She arranged for Daniel and his mother to come in for a visit so she could see for herself. When they arrived, she had him walk up and down the hallway to confirm that he still had the typical gait of a child with mild spastic hemiplegia. He did. Then she asked him to run. To her astonishment, he ran like a normal boy, with an easy, balanced stride and normal reciprocal arm movements. He performed tight pivot turns, at speed, on both legs. He could also turn at speed, then kick a soccer ball accurately with either leg. He performed perfectly when he was running.

After seeing this, Dr. Pape said, "You can't do that!" For the life of her, she could not figure out what was going on. We all know children learn to walk before they run. Yet here was a child who had turned conventional wisdom upside down. This set her on a path to study cerebral palsy and how the brain can heal. It ended up taking many years for Dr. Pape to realize that doctors' classical assumptions of permanent brain damage were wrong and Daniel's normal run meant that his brain had recovered from early injury. The damage had been repaired, or the brain had grown in its capacity to compensate. Or new neural pathways had been forged in his brain to get around the original damage. This was the beginning of her life's research into neuroplasticity.

Dr. Pape goes on in her book to describe classical doctors' reasoning for cerebral palsy. These doctors assert that the brain is rigid and therefore is hardwired and cannot change after brain damage. Over a lifetime of dedication and hard work, Dr. Pape proves this theory as flat-out wrong, and Dr. Norman Doidge reinforces it in his book, *The Brain That Changes Itself*. Our brains, especially those of babies and small children, can and do heal. This is called neuroplasticity and is the basic theory behind all the transformational breakthroughs throughout my entire life.

The good news is that neuroplasticity is not only found in babies and kids. This transformational plasticity is available for all of us, for our entire lives! However, many classically trained doctors tend to be of the "pill and drill" mentality. I should know because I have met quite a few over the years. All these doctors wanted to do was dope me up and drill on my back to fuse my vertebrae, or work on my legs to correct this or that, or operate on my foot to realign my toes instead of less invasive procedures. My parents ended up being my strongest advocates for alternatives to surgery. Only by a miracle did I not end up having more surgeries or medications prescribed throughout my life.

There are way too many stories in my history where doctors just wanted to pill me up and drill. There are less invasive ways to achieve proper mobility—less radical and less harmful ways. I have found that we must focus on retraining the brain to send correct neurological signals. How to send these signals more efficiently should be investigated and put into action first.

I often think of it this way: when you drive down a road and hit a pothole, you learn to avoid that pothole next time by maneuvering around it. With time, this becomes a habit. Then, let's say, one day the pothole is filled in during the dead of night, when no one sees that it has been filled in. You have learned to avoid that pothole, so you continue to go around it—a pothole that is no longer there. The pothole represents brain damage and the neuropathway to the body part you want to move. When your brain heals, it still thinks it should take that original, inefficient pathway around the pothole, or damaged area, called a neural circuit, to the body part it wants to move. We must retrain the body to use this new, efficient pathway that goes over the old pothole. This is what I have coined "brain–muscle alliance." The body's alliance between your brain and muscles—training and developing the muscles—is a transformational process that the body and brain will benefit from every time. Simply put, everyone does benefit from neuroplasticity. It's all in how to go about training the brain to be efficient in building good, strong neuromuscular memory pathways. Neuroscientists call muscle memory a "facilitated brain network,"[48] and they have been studying this fascinating field for years.

THE FOOT EPIPHANY

Another transformation epiphany hit me in early 2018, after nearly eight years of working with Ruth and thirty-four years of wearing doctor-pre-scribed custom arch support orthotics due to my flat feet and CP. One day on the workout floor, Ruth had me remove my shoes and realized I was wearing arch supports. Perplexed and a little excited, she wanted to attempt something new with me. She had me walk barefoot across the gym floor, noting how I walked. Then she had me perform several perfect full Olympic bar squats with two plates per side (225 total pounds). I was amazed that my knees stayed in perfect alignment, that my legs were working perfectly, my feet straight and heels digging in, with my toes lifting slightly off the ground with each squat. My body was, in fact, stronger without my shoes on. I was in proper alignment, and I was able to fully "feel" the floor with my feet without my shoes and orthotics getting in the way. But how was this possible?

Over the past years, the muscle growth and tone in my feet had strength-ened to the point where my hard, custom-fabricated orthotics were actually causing harm to my feet, which translated up my whole body to impede proper neurofeedback from "feeling the floor." This feat of action wasn't possible years ago, due to my toe misalignment and weak right foot, toe, and leg muscles. Over the years of intense training with Ruth, my right foot had gained muscles but still lacked proper neural signaling and feedback that the floor normally would have given me if not for my orthotics dampening this proper feedback. She said I no longer needed orthotics and that wearing them was restricting me from growing even stronger. I formally retired my arch supports on August 21, 2018, and it took me a while to adjust to feeling the floor with every step. Ruth even encouraged me to go barefoot as often as possible to further reinforce this new neurofeedback circuit. Today, while working out, I wear five-finger cross-training shoes on the workout floor, if not going barefooted altogether. Kinesiology-wise, the theory she was test-ing was that my brain needed the tactile neuro-responses from the ground to properly signal my leg and foot muscles. In layman's terms, I needed to be grounded and "feel the floor." I needed to feel the earth below me to perform these complex movements—a case in which being grounded is actually a positive experience (pun intended).

ONE STEP BACK, THREE STEPS FORWARD

Over the years, I have been told that being an athlete and bodybuilder would come with a few setbacks. I don't think this is necessarily a reliable forecast. Nonetheless, if you are smart about what you are doing, perform your tasks correctly, and train under expert supervision, you can minimize these setbacks.

On the surface, some setbacks can seem like just that: setbacks. However, when you dig deeper, some of these are really a reckoning to unexpected and unforeseen gains that may not have happened at all without a trigger event.

On December 10, 2018, while setting up for my assigned workout, I tripped into my first major setback, hearing a loud pop. It was one of those Monday mornings: the gym was overcrowded, and there seemed to be static in the air. You know the feeling, when everyone is trying to get their "skinny on" before the holidays. Not many workout spots were open, and it felt like nobody had much concern for anyone but themselves. I usually just tune everything out with my noise-canceling over-the-ear headphones playing Hillsong United or one of my other upbeat playlists, while reminding myself to stay humble and just concentrate on my workout. On this particular morning, I was at one of two Smith bar press stations. I had set up my station with an adjustable bench with wheels on one side and a handle for moving on the other. Everything was nice and tidy. As usual, I arranged my workout towel and iPad on the bench, with my workout routine displayed so I could record what I was doing and the weights I was using. I tested out the weight I had just added on the bar and adjusted the bench exactly right. Since I was going to combine two exercises, known as a superset, I was going to be pressing with another exercise that required dumbbells. I made my way through the jungle of folks to the free weights, grabbed my desired pair of dumbbells, then headed back to my little corner. To my surprise, a young lady had moved my bench with my iPad and towel on it out from under my Smith bar and was unsuccessfully attempting to unrack my weights. My humility was tested at this point as I engaged her in conversation.

"Ma'am, I am working out here," I said.

"I did not see that anyone was using this station," she replied in a snippy voice while looking at my bench with my stuff on it.

Humility was about to leave the building. "What part of all this stuff on this bench under that bar led you to that conclusion?" I retorted.

She took another look at the bench with my stuff on it, which she had just moved, and replied in an entitled manner, "You don't have to be so snotty about it," then walked to the very next unoccupied Smith bar press to begin her workout there.

At this point, I should have taken a mental timeout, checked my blood pressure, and called it quits. Inside, I felt like Jack Torrance, played by Jack Nicholson in *The Shining*, when he chops his way through the door with an ax, grins, and says, "Here's Johnny!"

I put my dumbbells down, removed my iPad and towel from my workout bench, and lifted the bench's handle to roll it back underneath my Smith bar, using a bit more force than I should have. The bench refused to move as I intended. The wheels did not go around and around, even when I put my might into forward motion, even leaning into it…and then, with a sudden, unexpected, and unwelcome release of the bench wheels, I felt a pop in my left arm. A pop so loud that I swear everyone must have heard it. The bench then started to move, and before I knew it, the bench was back under my bar. Not wanting my ego bruised from what sounded like the loudest pop I had ever heard in my life, I quickly took my position and hammered out a nice set, and then I got up to add more weight. It was only when I went to pick up a mere five-pound plate that I felt the sheer pain and lack of strength in my upper left arm. I almost dropped the weight in the process. My left biceps was on fire, and I had no supinated biceps strength at all. Game over! Grabbing my towel and iPad, I headed home for an ice pack.

I called Ruth that evening, letting her know that I thought I'd pulled a muscle in my left arm and that I had iced it down. She wanted to see me as soon as possible.

The very next day after work, when I arrived at her gym, she told me to warm up and she would take a look. Sonny Steppington, Ruth's assistant fitness manager, was the first to see me warming up on the floor. She immediately noticed that something was wrong with my left arm and shoulder… something terribly wrong. Slowly, these two trainers approached me with a look of genuine concern on their faces. A look that I had never seen on them before and one that I will remember for the rest of my life. I knew this was not a good sign.

After a quick evaluation and consultation between these two professionals, they agreed that I needed to go to the hospital right away and would likely require surgery. Okay, I thought, this sounded really bad. "But it's only a flesh wound," I wanted to say, but due to the seriousness in their tone, I knew better.

But where and how would all this go down? I thought. They recommended a facility right up the road called Direct Orthopedic Care. If I left right away, I might just make it before they closed at 6:00 p.m. So, at 5:40 p.m. I bolted out the door for the seven-mile drive in Austin rush-hour traffic to the doc's office.

"God, help me get there in time," I prayed as I negotiated traffic on south-bound IH35. Arriving at 5:58 p.m., I made a mad dash across the parking lot and "calmly" walked through the door of the doctor's office to a very cheerful and kind receptionist who greeted me with a "Wow, made it just in time" greeting.

I was checked in, evaluated, X-rayed, and consulted, all within forty-five minutes that evening. It felt like a full pit crew working double time during an Austin Formula 1 race. And to top it all off, I was going to be placed in an immobilized arm splint and scheduled for surgery that very next Monday. This splint would be my first splint ever worn for 24 hours a day on my left arm, and I had a lot of trouble getting used to having my dominant arm restrained in such a restrictive manner for an extended time. Throughout the whole series of procedures and evaluation, they kept asking me how much pain I was in, and I calmly reported "not much," as long as I did not use my left biceps. On a scale of 1 to 10, I reported a 2 and a 4 when I used the arm. The staff seemed perplexed at my report. Since it was late, Dr. Christopher Hall wanted to see me the very next day for a sonogram and MRI to confirm the extent of my injury.[49]

Oh boy! This was not the news I was hoping for.

Over the next day or two, Dr. Hall texted several times with various answers to questions I had, along with information including an animated YouTube video on the surgery he was going to perform. I must admit that this video was really cool and informative to watch. Dr. Hall's bedside manner and this information on the upcoming procedure helped soften my anxiety quite a bit. He also said that this type of injury was quite common among middle-aged, athletic bodybuilding males on their dominant side.

I replied, "Damn! You called me middle-aged," and I think he got a real kick out of that. He then replaced my shoulder-arm splint with an arm brace that kept my arm at a forty-five-degree max extension angle and my hand in a neutral thumbs-up position.

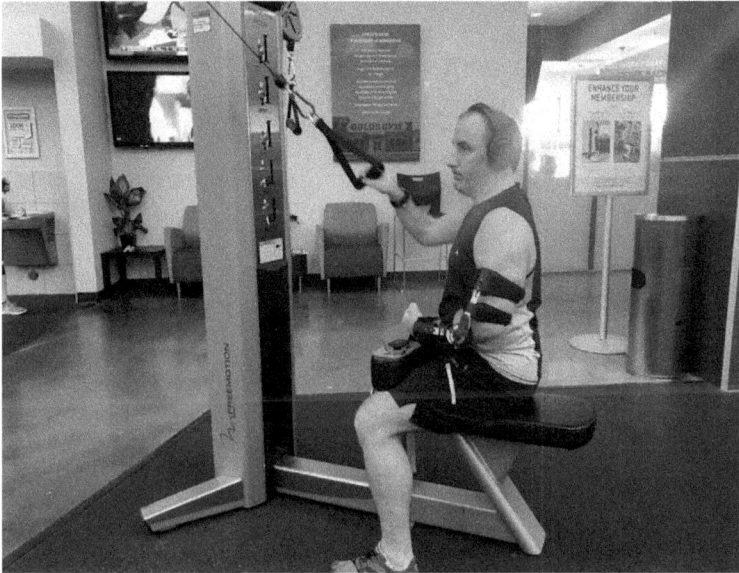

Working out right before left-arm biceps surgery

The day before surgery, while I was still in my arm brace, I went down to Gold's for one last workout before my surgery and long recovery were to begin. Dr. Hall said it was okay to do so, as long as I did not use my left arm in any way and remained in my brace. So I focused on my upper right-hand grip, arm-chest type movements with cable rows, and strong cardio. It felt good to be back on the gym floor.

Ruth called my mom during surgery to see how I was doing. She seemed genuinely concerned for my well-being and health. This gave me and my family great comfort.

Surgery went smoothly, and I was placed in a cast that immobilized my left wrist and forearm completely. I don't remember much of the next three days due to strong opioid-based painkillers and a nerve block that the doc had given me. After three days, I decided to stop the pain meds for the return of some sanity.

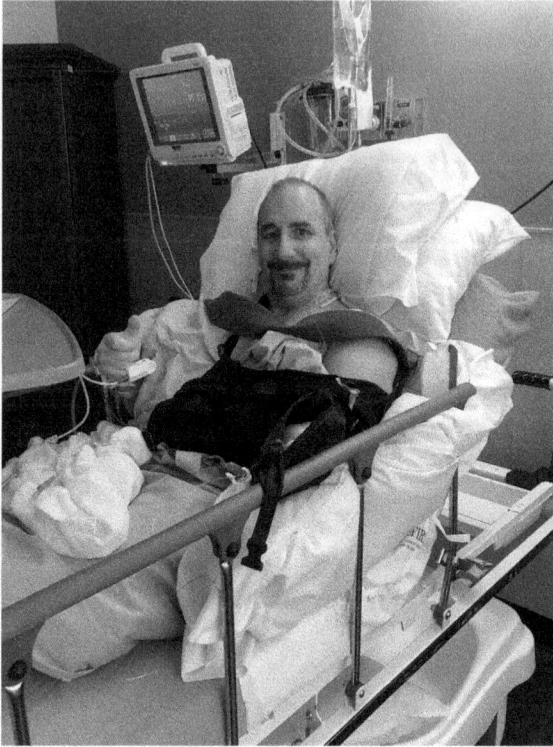

After left-arm surgery

Three long weeks went by. I had to learn how to perform everything with my right hand only, my CP-side hand, for the first time ever. Eating was one of the first challenges I had to conquer. Since spastic hemiplegia CP affects my entire right side, I had never developed the ability to hold a fork or spoon, much less a drink. Right-hand dexterity had not been one of my triumphs...until now.

Sometimes you must take a step backwards to move forward. In this case, I had crossed another threshold, another defining moment in my transformation: using my right hand and arm as my new dominant side, my *only* side at this point. There would be no cheating, either, since I literally had my left arm and hand tied up. I had to learn for the first time how to eat, shave, drink, and even shower this new way. Showering presented numerous challenges, starting with placing a plastic bag on my left casted arm. Sounds simple, right? Try placing a bag and rubber band on your dominant left arm with a right hand that tends to tactically rebel at every step. I became rather good at that as well as shampooing and washing my body using only my right hand. The hard part was hand-supine movements to hold the shampoo in my hand while moving quickly to my head before spilling my hand's contents on the floor for lack of rotational strength, keeping my right hand in a "bowl" position full of shampoo. Let's just say that a lot of shampoo never made it to my head in those early days. It wasn't graceful, but functionally it did the job.

Shaving presented a significant problem as well. Try lathering up and shaving with your nondominant side only. Then magnify that by a factor of a thousand, and you start to get into my realm of frustration. I started to lather up and shave right-handed only for the first week or so but found it too frustrating for lack of coordination and dexterity, plus the strength to hit all the unique angles a razor must contour. I decided it was time for a full beard, not just my traditional goatee.

As the weeks progressed, I learned how to do other things in unique ways as well. Driving a car right-handed had started several months prior, but I had always had a safety net then—that of my left hand at the ready. Now my right hand had to take over completely while my left hand sat uncomfortably in my lap, casted and braced, eager but unable to take over. Fastening my seatbelt using only my right hand was also impossible before this period. Known as one of the three proprioceptive neuromuscular facilitation (PNF) exercise patterns, a classical D2 shoulder flexion movement in the physical therapy world, I knew this movement as a long and drawn-out challenge. Fastening my seatbelt took well over ten tries at first. That final click, as my seatbelt secured itself into the latch, was a very welcoming sound and a relaxing feeling to my entire clenched body after each mini workout.

My new way of eating and drinking right-handed reminded me of what a two-year-old must feel like. These young ones crudely hold their utensil in a fist-like grip with an awkwardly bent wrist, scooping their food and lowering their head to meet their utensil. Yep, that was me: gripping my fork and spoon in a shovel-style ulnar-deviated-wrist fashion, scooping up my food, then ungracefully approaching my mouth in a maneuver that was both a race to see who would win (food to the floor or target reached at every bite), and a speed test to see how fast and steadily I could safely execute this maneuver. I think the floor won more than I reached the target in those early meal sessions. My emotions ranged from embarrassment and anger to fear of making a mess at every meal—and it was part of every meal experience for me at that time. As my recovery progressed, I became more like a four-year-old eater. Still messy but not as hungry. Drinking was a bit easier. I had learned to use an adult-style "sippy cup" with a straw and a base that had a suction cup, as I would lean over to drink. Again, it was functional but not very elegant. Needless to say, there were no formal black-tie dinner parties for Scott for the foreseeable future.

On December 31, I returned to my doctor's office for my first post-op follow-up. Dr. Hall was glad to see me. He cut off my cast and placed my arm in the X-ray machine at all sorts of angles, and then I waited for the buzzing of the X-ray machine and arm repositioning to end. He came in and asked me to bend my elbow and rotate my wrist in all sorts of strange ways. After noting a few things on his handheld tablet, he said that my recovery was going better than he had initially expected. I had far greater muscle tone than he anticipated and very little pain or inability to move. He said that usually they place their patients back into a new cast for another two to three weeks, but in my case, he wanted me to just wear my brace and move my arm as much as I could handle the pain. He prescribed no lifting, just movement. He wrote me a script so that I could resume my training with Ruth, but no left arm work at all.

I was so happy. After leaving the doctor's office, I headed straight for the gym where Ruth was working to tell everyone the great news and, of course, to work out. I was going back to the gym to continue my training! I did not have the nerve to reveal to my doc that I had already visited the gym on my own for light cardio and some right-arm work. After all, I knew I needed to condition my right side to step up my game.

Over the next six weeks, Ruth put together a plan with my doctor to further strengthen and accelerate my right-side potential, and I ate it up. I wanted more with every session. I learned how to do one-arm Smith bench presses at ground level and hold dumbbells and kettlebells right-handed only. My right side and core grew like never before. I could see my right forearm muscle growing bigger as my grip and wrist firmed up and straightened out. By forcing my right side to step up and take control, I was increasing the neuromuscular functioning on my right side faster than I would have on my present course before this tear.

Bring it on, I thought. On the inside I felt amazing!

On February 5, 2019, Dr. Hall cleared me to begin left biceps PT. I was so jazzed! Both he and Ruth said I would need to take it slow and steady and not rush it. No stopping me now! That first PT session consisted of baseline measurements and work to chart out my recovery. Lifting began with right-hand American and Russian kettlebell raises and five- and ten-pound left dumbbell curls in a supine standing position, ending with running on the treadmill at intervals of five, six, and seven miles per hour for three minutes. Superset two-minute walk, repeat with next speed up. Wearing my five-fingered workout shoes and my triathlete sport watch, I ran like never before.

"How do you feel?" Ruth asked.

"I feel amazing! Spectacular! Awesome! Fantastic! Wonderful!" I replied. God knew I could do more. I wanted more.

On March 7, 2019, I hit another milestone. I returned to my presurgery bench press max lifting weight. However, unlike before, I was able to bench-press with my right elbow in proper alignment, scapulars fully retracted, and my right wrist firm and straight—not bent backwards like before. My right wrist bending backwards was a classic CP trait that would cause pain and cause my right elbow to centralize or move in toward my rib cage for "protection," thus preventing my right scapula from fully retracting. By focusing on my right-side neuromuscular pathways and strengthening my right side, I was able to bring my right upper body into alignment with my left, thus achieving growth and strength moving forward. Now I could build both sides of my body together.

On March 27, 2019, Dr. Hall once again took X-rays and sonograms and evaluated me, then pronounced me fully cleared—fit to return to working out with my trainer without any restrictions. He said that I could progress in my training as tolerated, that my full recovery from biceps surgery was six months ahead of schedule, and that I had gladly proven him wrong on two fronts: one, my left biceps recovery had been remarkable and far greater and faster than he had expected or seen before, and two, my right arm with CP was far outpacing anything he had ever heard of. He attributed it to the aggressive conditioning work that Ruth and I had been pursuing since 2011.

Dr. Hall had first taken the stance that the neuromuscular "reeducation" process I was pursuing as part of this transformation would do little, if any, good when I first presented this plan to him. Now it seemed that he was incredibly pleased with my progression and transformation and was starting to rethink his stance on neuroplasticity altogether. They even printed my case and testimony as a success story in their bound case studies in their waiting rooms and on their website for doctors and clients to read.[50]

THE NEW NORMAL

Up to this point, I had been training as an athlete and bodybuilder for eight years. As I pen this book, I am still in a constant state of muscular, neurological, and attitudinal (proprioceptor) transformation. With what now seem like exponential changes accruing with every workout, I am constantly having to relearn what "normal" really is by the day. By this I mean what can I now do consciously and subconsciously to integrate these new movements and postures into my everyday life? Case in point: how I now use my right hand and arm is completely different from just three months ago. My left biceps surgery proved to me and many others just this point. I now have much better control of ROM and muscular neurological interaction than when I first began this transformation…and very often this catches me by surprise. How I walk, stand, and hold myself is a completely different "norm" than, say, two months ago, or even three weeks ago. I often surprise myself when seeing my reflection—not as in, "Damn, he looks good," but rather, "Wow, I am a completely different *me* than before!"

By this time in my transformation, Ruth (she was the fitness manager by this point) would make a special effort to introduce me to folks looking at joining as well as VIPs who would just "show up" at her gym. I began to feel important, like a rock star, whenever she introduced me to others and told of my CP and my transformation into the athlete standing in front of them. This positive reinforcement made it a lot easier for me to push harder, reach higher, and become stronger. The VIPs were intrigued and wanted to know more. They wanted to follow my journey. This was another incredibly strange but positive feeling for me. I had trouble feeling like a true athlete even though I was one now.

This feeling followed me onto the workout floor as well. On the floor, Ruth often reminded me that I could no longer trust how I "feel" while I am performing an exercise because often what feels wrong to me is actually what is correct for the very first time. Over time and training, it should soon become my new normal or what should "feel right." I often became aggravated at this seemingly controversial feeling because we all learn at an early age what normal positioning of our body is or how our body attitude is in relationship to its surroundings (proprioception).

This new movement or positioning that I am now performing just feels wrong to me. In the neurological world, the concept is explained this way: my proprioceptors, those nerve clusters that tell my brain where I am in relationship to the movements I am performing, have been "recalibrated" and are experiencing a new range of movement in terms of where I am in space and how my body is responding to that stimulus. This new normal is shifting by the day, and it's difficult to "trust" my feelings as to what is correct. Even looking in the mirror at my movements while weight lifting looks wrong. This is because, as much as I "trust" what my body looks like to me, these new movements often play tricks on my mind and convince me that something does not look right. This is another reason Ruth told me to put my brain in the locker and just do what she asked me to do.

Many breakthroughs now occur because I no longer have the old limitations of bad form or incorrect movements due to posture or limitations of my spastic cerebral palsy that once dominated my existence. Learning what this new normal is will be both challenging and exciting for what I (and others, through me) will be able to accomplish.

NEW "FIRSTS" AND ACHIEVEMENTS

Back in early 2014, Ruth wanted my help in creating an easy-to-use, real-time workout document to track my fitness progression. Since 2011, we had been utilizing the traditional Gold's Advanced Progress Chart that trainers would use with their clients. This paper chart card would be used on the floor to track progress and list out exercises the client would follow every week. It was becoming a bit overwhelming to track my progress, and I was starting to amass a large file cabinet full of these sheets. Since I would visit various other gyms across the city, I had to either take photocopies of these sheets prior to my assigned workout or call and have a staff member search for updates. We both realized the old way of doing things had to change; we needed a better way of tracking my progress in real time. I developed what became known as Scott's Transformation Workout Log and logged my first digital workout on November 10, 2014. This log was built utilizing an online platform so both of us could see and edit my workout progress in real time. I could follow while on the workout floor, and Ruth could assign "homework" and monitor my daily progress.

We originally only tracked workouts, status, and notes (such as reactions and how I felt, how my body responded), and traditional stats such as weights lifted and reps. There was also a tab for goals, both short-term and long-term.

In 2015, I amped it up a bit and redesigned the platform to be able to record statistics such as workout times and calories expended during a workout. Then by midyear, I added daily calories consumed and set points for calories for each day along with a color-coded dashboard for easy charting to my set goals and variances to these goals. It became my log for every workout, every day from that point on.

As an industrial systems engineer, I had learned that to achieve a goal, you first have to set goals, then place tolerances to these goals (upper and lower control limits) and measure progress to that goal. Since I also possess a master's in computer information systems, it seemed like a great idea to build a cloud-based training platform, which became my measuring stick from that point on. Today, I have added even more automation and other segments that record clinical data and other statistics to be used for fine-tuning progress in real time.

One segment of this transformation log lists out what I refer to as "my firsts." These are workout breakthroughs or "first-time events" that have occurred as a direct result of my transformation on and off the workout floor. These are tasks or achievements that had never been possible before my transformation began and may seem trivial to some. However, remembering that I have CP, which, at one time, limited my right side from a full *normal* potential, is simply amazing. The ability to have my body work in concert with each side is such a joy to experience. These "firsts" represent a huge neuromuscular gain, further proof that neuroplasticity does happen and can happen for anyone, regardless of their condition.

As I've established, I don't do "easy" very well. I go straight to "hard" and master it. A friend once told me that this determination to overcome the hard stuff in life is what truly makes me unique, and as I thought about that for a moment, I felt grateful. Throughout my childhood I had been afraid of failure, so I guess, on a subconscious level, I simply refused to play by the rules. I found the things that most people would consider difficult and strived to show them (and myself) what I could really accomplish.

Hope, positive thinking, sheer motivation, and a determination to excel are the prerequisites for great achievements to thrive.

Leo had surpassed all expectations; he may have been a late bloomer, but when he did bloom, it was indeed spectacular. And that timid mouse in Ruth's maze? Well, he grew into Mighty Mouse, then flew higher than anyone could have ever dreamed.

I went from a shy kid with CP to an athlete and bodybuilder who could now achieve these firsts, and what follows is a sample list of accomplishments, milestones, timelines, and recognitions, compiled from my journal and workout logs:

- January 12, 2011—Began training with Ruth King, priming for my transformation.

- May 1, 2012—Returned to restart transformation after a seven-month sabbatical in Colorado.

- Summer 2013—A surprise transformation recognition: showcased at the 2013 Gold's Gym leadership conference in Dallas, Texas, where general managers and trainers met with Executive VP of Fitness Tim Keightley for Gold's annual corporation meeting. One of two people singled out in the entire US.

- August 24, 2013—Completed 5K Color Run in Gunnison, Colorado, in fourth place.

- March 1, 2014—First time I was able to start a car right-handed.

- May 19, 2014—*Austin American-Statesman* featured my transformation story: "No More Limitations for Man with Cerebral Palsy."[51]

- December 16, 2014—Won Gold's transformation challenge, fall 2014 (West Lake Hills, Austin, Texas).

- June 2015—Shot Glock 19 handgun right-handed with same accuracy as left, dominant hand.

- August 5, 2015—Completed first unassisted bench press (forty-five-pound Olympic bar plus ten pounds).

- October 26, 2015—Started training with new trainer (Brian); transformation accelerated.

- December 31, 2015—Completed first unassisted dips (body weight).

- December 31, 2015—Did first full-body push-ups to the floor.

- May 8, 2016—Won second Gold's transformation challenge, spring 2016 (Hester's Crossing, Round Rock, Texas).

- January 26, 2018—Achieved first successful right-handed catch of a lacrosse ball.

- February 16, 2018—Full right-shoulder mobility scapula retracted without traps engaging.

- February 26, 2018—Completed first Olympic bar squat with two plates per side (225 total pounds).

- June 1, 2018—Did max T-bar row with four plates (180 pounds).

- June 7, 2018—Completed max dead lift lockouts of 315 pounds (six plates).

- August 21, 2018—No longer needed foot arch supports (started at fifteen years old).

- September 13, 2018—Developed a full six-pack (pictured on Wall of Fame).

- November 19, 2018—Completed first Olympic bar bench press with a plate, for a total of 135 pounds.

- December 10, 2018—Tore left biceps at insertion point forearm (a step back in training).

- December 17, 2018—Underwent left biceps surgery (arm in sling until March).

- January 1, 2019—Put on seatbelt with only my right hand for the first time.

- February 5, 2019—Doctor cleared me to begin left biceps PT.

- March 19, 2019—Doctor cleared me to resume bodybuilding six months earlier than expected.

- May 22, 2019—Won third Gold's transformation challenge, spring 2019 (North Round Rock, Round Rock, Texas).

- June 1, 2019—Completed bench press with right-hand knuckles aligned and wrist straight.

- June 3, 2019—The "reckoning" began (more on this later), severely limiting use of my dominant left arm.

- February 3, 2020—Had my first session with Brian Williams, began new records and challenges.

- February 15, 2020—Wrote right-handed for the first time (CP side).

- May 20, 2020—Consciously bent right toes for the first time (CP side).

- June 8, 2020—Balanced on my knees for the first time on a stability ball.

- June 17, 2020—Balanced on a stability ball while lifting weights.

…and more every day.

My transformation seemed to be back on track from my biceps tear, and I was experiencing new breakthroughs even more frequently than before. However, with a twist of fate, tragedy would come. Mighty Mouse's first flight led to hitting a wall and going into a tailspin, which led to a reckoning, soon to follow.

PART 8

The Reckoning

*There Is Another Way
When the Walls Are Closing In*

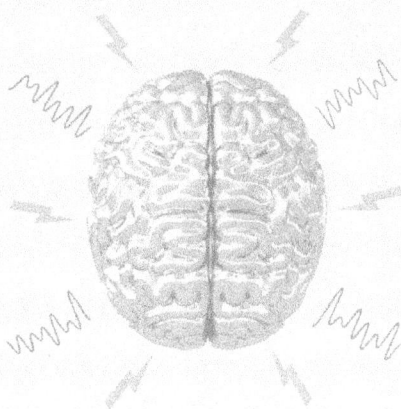

The Day the Reckoning Began

ON JUNE 3, 2019, EXACTLY TEN WEEKS FROM THE DAY THAT DR. HALL cleared me after biceps surgery, my life took an unexpected turn that cost me dearly.

There's a nautical term called *reckoning* that my friend Jimmy McNeil once explained to me—and it has stuck with me ever since. He explained that "reckoning" means making small changes or adjustments that can (and will) have a significant impact on one's trajectory over time. In my case, I am the vessel, and my trajectory is where I go from here.

In the weeks following that day, I kept hearing the word *reckoning* everywhere I went. Even though I was raised in a nautical family, it would take me several painful months to learn the real significance of this word in my life to come.

"Another in the Fire" is one of my favorite workout songs.[52] I had listened to this song during almost every workout, from the time it was first released. Sung by Hillsong United, from their 2019 album *People*, this song is about reckoning:

There's a grace when the heart is under fire

Another way when the walls are closing in

And when I look at the space between

Where I used to be and this reckoning

I know I will never be alone

* * *

There was another in the fire

Standing next to me

There was another in the waters

Holding back the seas

And should I ever need reminding

Of how I've been set free

There is a cross that bears the burden

Where another died for me

* * *

There is another in the fire...

It is known that God loves His children so much that, every now and then, He chooses to allow a slight course correction in their lives to keep them out of harm or from a possible destructive path that would or could ultimately follow. This was painfully revealed to me one Sunday morning at the Austin Stone Community Church, when Jimmy McNeal, our worship leader, took some time to fully explain a line of this song:

"When I look at the space between where I used to be and this reckoning…"

I had heard this line over and over again, but when Jimmy talked about the meaning behind this reckoning, it hit me like…well, like I had hit a wall at high speed. In fact, that's exactly what happened the evening of June 3, 2019. I hit a wall and went into a tailspin that I nearly did not recover from. This was the day my reckoning began, for I was set on a whole new unexpected trajectory that followed—the aftermath.

THE RETURN TO SKYDIVING WITH CEREBRAL PALSY—THIRTY YEARS LATER

During the early spring of 2019, while writing the story of my early years learning to skydive,[53] I met up with Keven Franks, an old friend who also went to college at Texas Tech. Although we did not meet while in college, he went through the same skydiving training during the same time period as I did. I wanted to get his valuable insights and feedback on the skydiving part of my manuscript. On May 22, 2019, Keven and I met at a somewhat secluded restaurant on the outdoor patio, where we could grab eats and drinks and not be disturbed. The events leading up to and including meeting at this place and time were way out of our normal routines. Our meeting on that back patio went well, with renewing old friendships, reviewing book content, reliving fond memories, and sharing our videos of skydiving. It was a fun time reconnecting.

I had never believed in chance or happenstance—some may even call it luck. Destiny has a way of showing up in the most unexpected places. That day on that quiet patio, as we discussed my story of skydiving, at the table right behind us sat a fellow enjoying a quiet evening with one of his favorite bottles of wine. Like us, he chose his table to be away from the crowd and escape the busyness of the evening. It was a typical Wednesday evening for him, a night to mind his own business and enjoy the quiet. But as he would tell us later, he kept hearing the word *skydiving* popping up from the very next table, and after the third time hearing it, he felt he had to introduce himself.

"Hello," he said. "I couldn't help but overhear you mention skydiving." Keven and I both turned around and introduced ourselves, and I gave a very abridged version of having cerebral palsy and working on a project including a book about neuroplasticity and my transformation.

"I am Steve Lively. How would you like a new ending to the skydiving chapter of your story?" he said.

Keven and I looked at each other, and our eyes probably gave us away. *Who is this guy? Some weekend tandem skydiving dude? Is he for real?* But after further dialogue, we discovered that Steve was a nationally ranked competitive formation skydiver based in the Greater Austin area and was very well known around those parts.

"I was intrigued by your conversation, and when you mentioned skydiving three times, just like Beetlejuice, I had to interject," he told us. "From what I overheard, you had some trouble with learning to skydive back in college. Now that you have a 'transformed body,' there should be no problem skydiving with CP. I can help lead you in your quest and even to certification. I know the best skydiving trainers in the business," he added.

Over the next couple of weeks, Steve and I ended up speaking about skydiving programs and the best way to proceed. I told him I was concerned about the CP limitations of my past, citing the issues I had experienced back in college with not being able to hold on with my right hand, and I also mentioned that my right arm was not as strong or as straight as my left. Steve reassured me that the instructor he wanted to introduce me to would know how to train me safely, even with my CP. These professional trainers at the local skydiving tunnel had trained folks just like me with CP, he added. He wanted to make a few calls and introduce me to one of the best instructors, who would love to come alongside and teach me the skills, process, and movements that I needed to master to become a successful skydiver. It seemed like CP would no longer prevent me from achieving the dream I'd had since my first solo jump thirty years prior.

A few weeks later, I met Steve once again at that same restaurant. We spoke about skydiving topics, and he invited me to an indoor skydiving tunnel located nearby, where I could meet the gang and get involved with the skydiving community. Steve told me that the instructor he had in mind would take all necessary precautions to keep me safe. He had talked with him and thoroughly explained my condition. He said that since I had CP, there should be two trainers, one on each side of me, and that he recommended they place me on my belly on the floor, then spin the tunnel up, so I would lift off the ground. They would proceed to teach me the necessary skills while keeping control of me at every stage of my training. Nervously, I took Steve up on his offer to meet Darrell Wong after my scheduled workout session with Ruth. I was nervous but also very excited.

I had been to this tunnel a couple of times before, just to watch friends on a flight or two, but had not wanted to do this myself. Not because I was scared. I just did not see the point or purpose…until now.

After I had hung around the tunnel for close to four hours, Steve introduced me to Darrell and others in this skydiving clan. Steve asked Darrell to be my instructor and lead me back into the world above, or at least that was the intention. Upon meeting me and getting to know my story, including fully understanding my limitations, the group seemed quite interested in helping me. I told Darrell I was extremely uneasy, but he reassured me that he would take extra-special care of all aspects of my training. At a local restaurant next to the tunnel, I showed Darrell and the gang my skydiving logbook and a video of me skydiving thirty years before. I described how the limitations on my right side led to overcompensation of my left side and how that had prevented me from continuing this training.

He asked me to reach up as high as I could, then back as far behind my back as I could, with both arms, to verify the range of motion that I had described. My right arm was not as straight or graceful as my left, and he took note of this. He said that it looked like I could still reach the parachute toggles fine, but we would have to work on the finer motions in the tunnel first. There was such an amazement and fascination from the group about my transformation and overcoming CP. It felt electrifying, and they were all jazzed about being a part of my story of getting back into skydiving.

"This is going to be fun, and we want to help document this journey to bring you airborne once again," Darrell said. "We will even film you for your book and everything." We talked about right versus left parachutic pulls and my limitations with deploying the "rip cord" using my right hand. "It is best that you stay with a left-pull procedure for now," he said, "since this side is your dominant side and has the most ingrained muscle memory." He added that he now had to pull his parachute left-handed too because he had broken his right shoulder in a tunnel accident a while back and could no longer pull right-handed. He showed me the surgical scar. It was long and right below his right shoulder. I told him I did not want one of those. He laughed and agreed.

"Once you get several jumps under you, we can work on throwing right-handed," he added.

"I am all for that," I replied.

Darrell then added, "You've already started on this journey and need only twenty-three more jumps to go."

With a perplexed look, I said, "Already started?"

"Yes. You have two jumps already, from 1990. These jumps here in your logbook count. Only twenty-three more to go. Let's get you into the tunnel," Darrell said. "How about we schedule time in the tunnel on Monday at 5:00 p.m.?"

This last question was one I wish I had said no to from the get-go and would later regret answering at all.

BLACK SWAN EVENT—HITTING THE WALL AT 1:43

The big evening had arrived. Steve and Ruth were unable to join me that evening, so I went alone. Darrell had told me not to wear my corrective lenses to the tunnel, as the wind in the tunnel would rip them right off. About ten minutes before the flight, I was told to rush downstairs, pay, and sign in. They wanted me to sign some paperwork on a tiny screen affixed to the wall. I tried to read all the small print, and when I asked for a printed copy, the attendant seemed to think it was funny and said they did not have the ability to print anything.

Darrell said I would be late if I did not hurry, so I reluctantly signed based on a verbal agreement that Darrell and his tunnel team would take extra precautions to ensure my safety. It was almost past time to suit me up, so I had to rush through a quick video on what was about to happen. I felt like I had ADD; all the new stimuli were overwhelming, and things were happening fast. Was I ready to learn to fly?

I was the first one in. The tunnel fired up, and the roar of the fan far below us sounded like a jet plane about to take off, loud, with a wind speed registering at 130 miles per hour. When Darrell and I entered the chamber, I was surprised to see that he was the only one in there with me. Where was the other guy? They had assured me there would be two. And why was the tunnel on already? Before I even realized what was happening, I was in Darrell's arms as he laid me onto the air stream. Everything felt strange but stable, even though my heart was racing at rocket speed. I was nervous—I had never done anything like this tunnel thing before—but I figured I could trust my instructor.

An incredible amount of overstimulation and a feeling of uneasiness was now rushing by me at over 130 miles per hour. Darrell backed away and motioned to me to spin.

How do I do that? I thought. After mere seconds that felt like an eternity, my body started to spin clockwise. How, I did not yet understand. Then all hell broke loose. One minute and forty-three seconds into my very first tunnel flight, my body spun fast and out of control, and my head and left arm slammed into the transparent cylindrical wall of the chamber at high speed, my left arm hyperextending over my head.

In that moment, I had no idea just how bad the hit really was. I was running on pure adrenaline, in literal fight-or-flight mode, and did not feel anything at that point. Darrell tended to another student, a very young kid who had seen me hit the wall and was too scared to enter the tunnel at all. I will never forget the look of sheer terror on the kid's face as he was led into the chamber. He kept looking at me as if I could help him somehow. He did not enjoy his flight and refused to go again. And before I knew it, Darrell was back to rush me through the process once again. I was later told that I flew for over nine minutes total.

It was only after I exited the chamber area and started to leave for home that I realized something was seriously wrong. As the adrenaline wore off, I could not use my left arm at all. I sat in my car wondering what to do. *Houston, we have a problem.* Darrell said I should have pushed off the wall and that the collision was my fault. "Shrug it off," he said. "You'll be okay." He didn't seem concerned at all. With my left arm rendered useless, I managed to drive home, in severe pain, using only my right CP-side arm.

That night was excruciating, and I did not get any sleep. The next morning, Tuesday June 4, I took the day off work, and at 9:00 a.m., Dr. Hall, my orthopedic doctor and surgeon, confirmed my worst fear. MRI scans showed that I had dislocated my left shoulder and torn my subscapularis and biceps tendon. I would require left-shoulder surgery ASAP.

I must have reviewed the video of my flight a million times, wondering how all this could have happened. Where was my trusted instructor? Where were the promised safety procedures for folks with CP? A thousand questions ran through my mind about how wrong the whole thing was.

I underwent shoulder surgery on June 13, 2019.[54] There was extensive damage, and it took well over four hours for my doctor and his team to complete the operation. This time, unlike with my previous surgery, Ruth did not call, text, or otherwise inquire about my health or well-being. I asked Mom after surgery if she had called like before. But to our surprise, no call or checkup from Ruth would come from that point on.

I soon began slow and steady rehab with an in-house physical therapist, on strict doctor's orders, with my arm in a braced, restricted sling all over again.

Seven weeks later, I had to return to Dr. Hall's operating table once more for revision surgery due to a complication with the healing process in my shoulder. More sonograms and MRIs confirmed that, sometime during weeks three and five of my recovery, the sutures binding my subscapularis tendon to my shoulder had not held, and the tendon was once again slowly tearing loose. My doctor said that as a result, the tendon was slowly receding down my back, and that was what was causing extensive pain between my shoulder blades (scapulae).

For the third time in seven months, I headed back into surgery. My third surgery was performed on August 1, 2019. This revision surgery was even more complicated than before. Dr. Hall spent over an hour just locating my subscapularis tendon, which had retracted four centimeters and was extremely hard for him and his team to reattach. Surgery lasted over four hours and took a total of seven anchors and three sutures per anchor to fully restore my shoulder once again.

Nine years of training, bodybuilding with my good friend and mentor as a trainer, the dream of ever skydiving again, and even writing this book, all came crashing to a halt, possibly even to an end.

My left arm was once again useless and back in a totally restrictive sling, and I had to rely solely on my CP arm and hand for everything. No more training, no more workouts, and no more profound transformation with Ruth coaching and training me. All I had to look forward to was lots and lots of pain, medications, and rehab. And I no longer had an athletic trainer to help me through this critical period.

This seemed to be my new life. What was once obtainable was now once again unattainable. I had hit a wall and had come crashing down, hard and fast.

LOSING MY TRAINER

As I mentioned, Ruth did not call or make any attempts to contact me or my family. No contact at all. It was as if she left me to hit another wall, a wall of abandonment. Ruth had set me on a path for great gains eight years prior, had built up my confidence, and had shown me what I could accomplish. And now, it seemed, I was no longer worthy of her attention. Bam! A second hit. She just left. She had played such a huge part in my life, and it seemed bizarre that she would just ghost me. No communication, not even a goodbye. By her inaction, she communicated that we were done, and I received the message loud and clear. It now seemed that I was in for one hell of a tailspin.

I don't know why Ruth abruptly ended all communication, especially at this critical point in my recovery and ongoing transformation. When professional athletes injure themselves during a sporting event, their training and support team rallies around them to get them back into the game. But I was not a professional athlete. In fact, I was just then learning how to perform as an athlete, both psychologically and physiologically. Over those eight years, Ruth had *finally* broken through my deeply ingrained childhood flight response and taught me how to build a healthy fight response as a highly tuned athlete. But now, when I needed a support system more than ever, I was left with a mind full of doubt, lots of regret, and questions I could not answer on my own. Ruth's refusal to communicate made these doubts, regrets, and questions grow bigger as the months and years of rehab progressed. My training support team was no longer there to help me heal and get back into the game.

I would have to find a new trainer, someone with not only the right credentials and experience training someone like me but someone who could also motivate and push me beyond my self-imposed limitations. I knew this would be difficult even without the added constraints of a complex injury, but in my current state, it seemed nearly impossible. I had lost a trusted advocate and had to fight my old tendency toward flight, toward returning to my old, "safe" ways that would ultimately mean no more athletic training or bodybuilding.

I had so many questions. Had Ruth grown tired of me? Was she unable to keep up with what she had created in me? Was I now too far outside of her wheelhouse of knowledge and understanding? I was no longer able to train, and she would no longer make any money off me—was this why she had disappeared?

Then my mind went off on another tangent: Was Ruth frightened that she had encouraged me to go too far "beyond my limits" as an athlete with CP? I had been injured twice and required three surgeries, and I might never be able to come back after the latest injury. Was she feeling some sort of guilt that I was injured multiple times on her watch? Or perhaps there was a deeper, more sinister reason, some sort of gag order imposed by someone who had prevented her from continuing as my trainer due to the nature or circumstances of my injuries. I would likely never know. I was alone, with very few athletic-minded professionals around to help keep my mind from going off on these unproductive tangents. For years, I was bombarded with these types of thoughts. These thoughts and many more tore at my mind after that night of my reckoning.

From my perspective, Darrell Wong, who had done very little, if anything, to prevent me from colliding with the wall and falling to the ground while under his care as a trainer, broke more in me than just the ligaments and tendons in my left shoulder. He broke my spirit of trust for professionals who are there to teach and train students in a safe, controlled manner. Ruth King, who had once unlocked my potential on the workout floor and beyond, had now left me to fall back into the very same box she had helped me out of years ago. By walking away, Ruth only reinforced the idea that I should not trust professional trainers because when times get rough, they will fail and let me fall.

The impact from these two inactions became a critical point of reflection in my transformation and recovery. I needed help. Faith had gotten me past some crazy things in my past, so I knew I had to look up and once again have faith that I would make it through this reckoning as well. I was at a crossroads: I could either fall back into the box of "you can't do that" that had governed my life with CP for so long, or I could resolve to never get back into that box ever again. I needed to look for the joy in all this so that faith would ultimately lead to perseverance. The choice was simple. I was never going to get back into that box, or any other box, for that matter!

PERSONAL TASKS IN A WHOLE NEW LIGHT

People have often asked me how I handled personal tasks during the twenty-eight-plus weeks of left-arm immobilization. Tasks like bathing and bathroom duties, for instance. Well, showering and bathing were exceedingly difficult at first, due to the haste of carefully removing my brace, to shower or clean and redress my wounds. This daily activity was painful and time-consuming for many months that followed. My right hand had to do all the work. Lifting my left arm was impossible due to the muscle and nerve damage from the incident and ensuing surgeries, so the engineer in me took over and devised several bathing aids that I rigged so that my right hand could effectively wash most of my body parts. This included string-pulley systems with sponges that I would hold and pull to manipulate for areas my left hand normally would have been able to handle.

These pulley systems reminded me of how it must have been for Dr. Emmett Brown to construct devices to feed his pet sheepdog, Einstein (or Copernicus) in the *Back to the Future* movies (portrayed by Tiger in the first film and Freddie in the other two).

I employed other innovative approaches in the bathroom as well, such as installing a bidet prior to surgery (insert blushing here), which would also bode well later, during the great COVID-19 toilet paper shortage of 2020. God is great and prepares His children well!

THE LONG ROAD CALLED PHYSICAL THERAPY

During the long months that turned into years, my recovery from the skydiving accident progressed slowly due to the nature of my surgeries and having to start all over for a third time in such a short time span.[55] Dr. Hall's approach and protocols for both shoulder rehabs called for extremely conservative rehab progression, the same protocol that is prescribed for a complete rotator cuff replacement. By the third time, I was gun-shy about any type of physical therapy treatment at all. My trust factor was being severely challenged. I could no longer work out, in the gym or otherwise. I continued to feel betrayed and totally alone. And like so many other folks with CP who get taught at an early age that they'll never be able to do this or that, I was beginning to think this way again. The sad fact is that I *had* done the things they said I could not do—I had done even more. But that was before it was all taken away in an accident that should have never happened. Before the reckoning.

Now deeply recessed memories resurfaced once more: memories of a small, shy boy with CP being told *no*, that I was not worth the effort. *Who was I to think I could be an athlete or bodybuilder with cerebral palsy? Why did I think I could learn to skydive with CP? I don't belong on the workout floor or in a wind tunnel chamber learning how to fly!* I thought. This inner voice would taunt me every time I went to rehab or saw skydiving videos on CHIVE TV.

However, I was more determined than ever before to flex my newly formed neural pathways and show that I had even more determination and persistence to stand back up and learn how to fly all over again—even if it took three attempts to do so. My old friends Determination and Persistence were back! From the very moment I entered the world, these playmates had accompanied me, and they were bolder than ever before, motivating me forward in this reckoning and recovery.

A TICKING BOMB—FRUSTRATIONS LIVING WITH CP

People who do not have CP will never fully understand what we go through. Heck, I have CP, and I am just now starting to understand what I've gone through, especially during these last few years. It is hard to put into words. People, in general, can have frustrations with their bodies not performing correctly, and those frustrations can run deep. Most "normal" able-bodied kids, however, learn how to express and overcome these frustrations early in childhood, perhaps badly at first, such as throwing temper tantrums. But later, they are able to express themselves and work through frustrations to understand what their bodies can do and how to achieve desired outcomes. With the neurological complications of cerebral palsy or stroke, however, this pattern of understanding, unless actively addressed, may never fully mature. What I mean is that when our bodies don't move or react in the way we expect them to, it affects us deeply, and we may not react well or predictably by these "normal" patterns in life. We have an awfully hard time processing these conflicts, and if not dealt with properly, unchecked frustration can lead to bad things. Today, we are finally beginning to understand more about CP.

Case in point, over the past eight years, I have made huge gains in my neuromuscular system known as brain muscle maps.[56] As I researched this brain-muscle-mapping concept, I learned that Dr. Wilder Penfield was the first neurosurgeon to have mapped a patient's brain. This involved determining what parts of the brain represented different parts of the body and processed their activities.[57] Today, we can see this through functional MRI (fMRI) scans. If I had been fortunate enough to have undergone fMRIs of the muscular control centers in my brain back in 2011, these maps would have shown significant changes (a.k.a. improvements) from then to now. Learning what my new "normal" was supposed to feel like now was tough since these changes were occurring so fast that my conscious mind had trouble keeping up with my brain-remapping currently in progress.

Experiencing multiple injuries from a catastrophic incident that resulted in the loss of the use of my dominant side altered these brain muscle maps even more. In fact, these changes radically occurred over the last nine months from my injury! That's a lot for any athlete to endure with some sense of clarity, much less an athlete with cerebral palsy. I was already having a hard time understanding what was going on and why all this was happening during my transformation and development of new muscles and abilities. Then, a triple whammy: three injuries requiring surgeries over a short period of time and extensive rehab thereafter. It was a huge source of internal frustration.

By this time, the pot was starting to boil. More to the point, I had a difficult time knowing what I should and should not be doing because of these sports-related injuries. How did professional athletes handle this process? Most likely, they'd have a staff of "experts" to help them through the intense mental and physical stressors associated with their performance and healing from their injuries. I did not have such experts to help me through the process of coping with these stressors. After all, my trainers and the folks who had motivated me to excel had all checked out of my life shortly before or after the reckoning had begun. So the stressors festered and grew. The pot boiled over with such voracity that everyone in the sports-segment part of my life split—like a hydrogen atom splitting at an atomic bomb party.

But I had no idea the bomb was ticking…or that there even was a bomb. I was just trying to understand and process these new experiences. My trainer up to this point had been highly successful in "getting me out of my own head" through various methods, like running laps, as I mentioned earlier. After all, she had to build that "fight" response in me when my natural tendency had been to take flight and give up before attempting to do anything. *Now* the frustration was building, and I was digging in and attempting to fight even harder through the storm. This was perhaps not the proper response to this kind of frustration, but I didn't realize it until slightly before the reckoning had begun. As a professional, my trainer should have seen this and perhaps had me "stand down" instead of fighting through the barrage of conflicts. Now, nine months after the reckoning began, I was just starting the long process of comprehending what had happened and how complex this process of *transformation* really is. Every day since hitting the wall has been a mental struggle to go on. I am in flight mode one day, then fight mode the next.

Ruth's mysterious departure turned up the flame of that that boiling pot. How such a small thing like unchecked frustration can exert so much force is astounding to me. Why did I not see this before now? Why did my former trainer not see it building? Or did she see it and refuse to act? All good questions that I hope will be answered as recovery and healing continue. It is my hope that you, the reader, will be able to recognize the same patterns before it's too late for others with CP or stroke who are in the process of building their own transformations.

Everyone hits a wall at some point in their growth. It's how we manage to pick ourselves back up that ultimately defines us. My reckoning had officially begun, and the aftermath was upon me.

THE HAWTHORNE EFFECT

In the aftermath of the reckoning, I was searching for answers to so many questions. In those early days of my transformation, Ruth had unlocked a potential energy source in me that ignited a far greater kinetic counterpart than anyone could have imagined or hoped for. And once I had learned that I could raise "the bar," I wanted to see how far I could push it, to "fly" to new heights. But as everything seemed to fall apart around me, I had to wonder, had I reached too far, too high? And why would the very person who championed my transformation disappear like a warp-drive starship leaving orbit?

As young kids, we look to our parents: "Daddy, Daddy" or "Mommy, Mommy, look at me!" And then we celebrate achievements in life together. Was there a subconscious parallel at play in the way I had always wanted to impress my trainer as I pushed and grew in new ways? Or did the drive to do more, the desire to achieve more, lead me forward without proper checks and balances that perhaps a trainer should have put in place? What had led me to this wall? Could it be that I was suffering from the Hawthorne effect?

The Hawthorne effect refers to the way in which people will modify their behavior simply because they are being observed or watched. This effect gets its name from one of the most famous industrial history experiments that took place at Western Electric's factory in the Hawthorne area of Chicago in the late 1920s to early 1930s.

The Hawthorne experiments were originally designed by the National Research Council to study the effect of shop-floor lighting on workers' productivity at a telephone factory.[58] The researchers were perplexed to find that productivity improved not just when the lighting was raised but also when the lighting was dimmed. Productivity also improved whenever changes were made in other variables such as rest breaks and working and nonworking hours.

The researchers concluded that the workers' productivity was not being affected by the changes in working conditions but rather by the fact that people studying them were concerned enough about their well-being and effort in conducting these experiments.

In my case, was I "producing better results" because I was being watched, tracked, and coached? Did I want to please my trainer more because I was the focus point? Like the maze scenario I presented earlier, Mighty Mouse knew the response/reward he would get because he was being watched, and Mighty Mouse wanted to fly higher for that reward. Did this lead to Mighty Mouse needing a new maze faster than the maze builder could build? Or was the maze builder tired of keeping up with the mouse altogether? Causality seemed to have been turned upside down. All I knew was that the wall was not the limit of my transformation potential—it was just a realignment point toward a new way of continuing with my transformation.

PART 9

The Recovery

Faith through the Fire

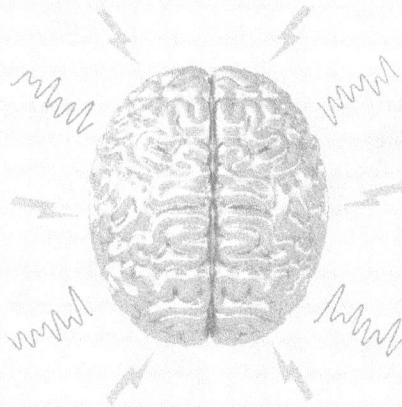

The Aftermath, Rehab, and the Pain

THOUGHTS OF DEFEAT REVERBERATED LOUDLY IN MY HEAD. *I AM DONE with this experiment. Never again will I let anyone convince me that I am able to do something like this. I am such a failure.* I wanted to quit, like my trainer had done with me. *I have CP. I can't do it. I reached way too high, and I fell.*

But something powerful was pushing me to press on and lean on Him. Lean and press hard! Something deep inside of me, pushing me, moving me in ways I thought I'd never want to explore again, ever!

By my third time in the operating room in less than a year, I was well known. In fact, one of my caretakers remarked that I should have a wing named after me for being a frequent flyer. The double pun was not lost on me (wing/arm…flying/skydiving). My response was that I would settle for a new wing (repaired shoulder) and let it be.

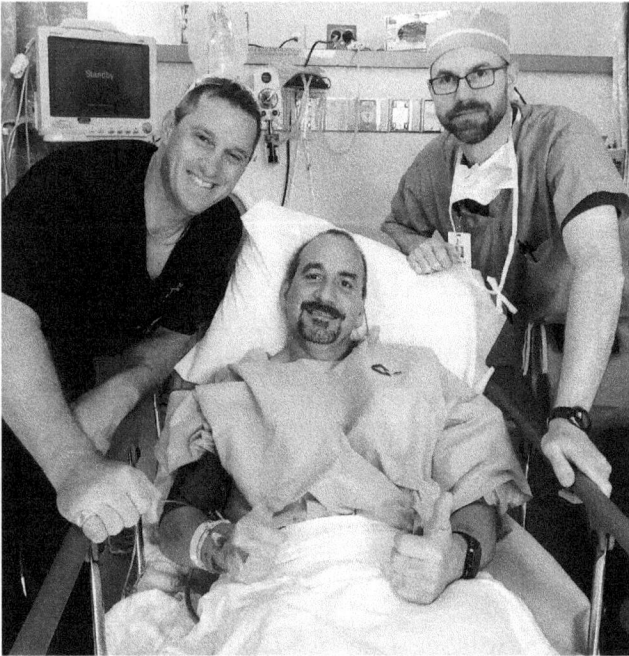

With my doctors right before shoulder surgery

I endured three hits as a result of hitting that wall on June 3, 2019: the *actual physical hit* from this trainer-led skydiving session, the *emotional hit*, and the *financial hit* that soon followed. Both the physical hit and resulting body damage were obvious to me now, and I knew that full recovery would take many years, if a full recovery was even possible. The emotional hit, I was just now starting to feel, and it seemed it might take even longer to heal than the physical.

The third hit was one that I was not at all prepared for. This hit seemed to be even harder to deal with, and it created more pain and suffering than either of the two hits mentioned above. Even before my surgeries began, I started receiving bills. I was contacted to pay for surgeries that had not yet taken place. If I did not pay, they would cancel my procedures. Then, about a month after the surgeries, I started receiving bills from all sorts of medical services, subservices, and my insurance company. They just kept coming from everywhere. My insurance company was fighting hard not to pay what they owed, and the hospital bills were more than the insurance company's rates of acceptance. My total portion of the bills was piling up fast. My "out of pocket" total was hundreds of thousands and growing by the month. This added even more stress to my pain, and unlike rehab, it was not getting better. To this day, I still get nervous when I open my mailbox, for fear of receiving yet another surprise medical bill. Amidst all this impact of recent events and tenuous financials, I was in jeopardy, with no possibility of a successful retirement at any time.

By hitting the wall, I was forced to fall back and reevaluate everything I was doing. My whole plan—my transformation, learning to skydive, weight lifting, training with a current or any future personal trainers, bodybuilding, and even writing this book—was in jeopardy of loss or remaining incomplete. Only many weeks later did I begin to realize what that initial whisper was really saying…it was saying I needed to completely lean on Christ and not my own understanding. I needed to remember that He is with me through this pain and suffering. I was now *in the fire with another standing next to me*, as the Hillsong United lyrics had so often told me.

SILVER LINING—USE IT, STRENGTHEN IT

From the aftermath of a biceps repair and two subscapularis surgeries on my left arm and shoulder in a seven-month period, I painfully came to realize that I had years of rehab and recovery to look forward to—much longer than I would ever have imagined. Whenever preventable incidents occur, such as what I had been through, one can look at them in one of two ways. You can either look inward to the misery and hurt, or upward, making the best out of a bad situation that you have been subjected to. I choose to always look upward, to see the light through the darkness. Some call this positive thinking; I call it being led by the light through the darkness.

"But when we humbly ask God to change us and empower us according to His will and His Spirit, it becomes transformational, and it glorifies God."[59]

—Brandon Zieske, Austin Oaks Church, 2020

Learning how to do everything with the nondominant side of your body is difficult enough for a "normal" individual. Combine that with having cerebral palsy on the nondominant side, and my transformation and recovery are truly amazing. As it turns out, this is a testament and strong case for neuroplasticity in real-life action.

MY FIRST POST-SURGERY SESSION

That first cardio rehab workout session was extremely hard and painful, and I had trouble plugging myself back into the music. With Hillsong United playing, I turned up the volume extra high to drown out that loud inner voice of defeat and begin once more. Five minutes…ten minutes…then fifteen. "I can do this," I kept repeating as "Another in the Fire" played deep within me.

That first workout ended up being one of the hardest things I have ever done. Tears ran down my face, painful and stinging sweat dripped down over my broken body—over my post-surgery pinned left arm. My body was slowly coming back online as the medications slowly filtered out of me. I kept repeating, "God, I know that with your strength in me, I will do this." One step at a time.

Faster and faster, I began to move on that Octane Fitness lateral slide cardio machine until I reached my desired cadence once again. Now to put this on auto drive and let Him continue to work in me. With my left arm in a sling pinned to my body and my right arm at my side, I began to energize and reestablish those old neuromuscular patterns once again as I listened to my music. After all, "neurons that fire together pair together."[60] Slow and uneasy at first, I was beginning to remember what job my core was to do. Step after step, stride after stride, I was starting to move once again. Before long, I even started to use my right hand, with CP, to reach, grab, and pull/push on the handlebar while my left remained in its sling, snugly strapped at my side.

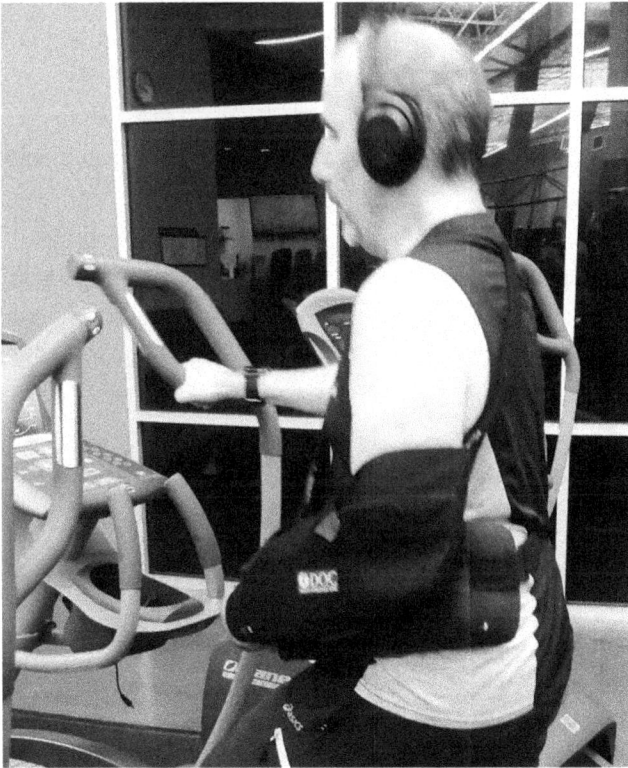

First workout after shoulder surgery, with pinned arm

Over the many months that followed, my right arm and right-hand grip became stronger and less sensitive and were now becoming the sole provider of grasp and grip. With every changing angle of my grip, I was adapting and growing muscles on my right side faster than ever before.

Out of necessity of survival, like learning to drive only right-handed, I was adapting to use my right side for everything. This process of adaptation was something that I never could have done before. Friends once again began to think that maybe all this kinesiology-neuroplasticity I had been talking about for nine years really did work. I was becoming a model of proof to my theories. It was no longer just something that I had been reading about, studying about, or talking about. I was transforming right out of the very pages of Dr. Karen Pape's book...or a personal triumph story that could be found in Dr. Norman Doidge's *The Brain That Changes Itself.* I was beginning to live out my own true success story in the making.

But could I really recover from this wall? Was recovery sustainable?

While at a gym far away from where Ruth and I once celebrated hitting new highs together (it was way too painful to ever return to Ruth's gym), in a full arm-immobilization brace, performing the only thing I had been cleared to do at that point—nonimpact cardio—I was often confronted by folks who would ask, "Rotator cuff surgery?"

"Yes," I'd respond. "Twice in seven weeks, in fact."

This ended up sparking a deeper conversation, which usually included them asking, "You really think doing cardio so soon is a good idea?"

Holding back internal sobs and tears, my response was, "Yes, I've got to keep moving forward even though I can barely crawl at this point." Deep down, I think it was really more about keeping myself from fleeing and never returning to this place of transformation ever again.

At this point in the conversation, I would usually let the proverbial cat out of the bag by revealing that I also had cerebral palsy on my right side. This news usually took a few seconds to really sink in:

Arm in brace on left side...CP in arm and leg on right side...

And then it would hit them like a bullet train at high speed, and *bang*, their eyes would light up with captivation and awe.

The first question after this was usually something like, "How do you manage?"

CONSTRAINT-INDUCED MOVEMENT THERAPY IN PRACTICE

Those who have had rotator cuff surgery know you must rely on your less-dominant side (usually) to support all daily activities, but having to rely on a "weaker," less-developed side with cerebral palsy is a concept that most people can't even fathom. But I can fathom it, all right. In fact, I have learned to welcome it as a greater sign of His strength in me. A true litmus test and proving ground for this whole concept of neuroplasticity and a strong motivator in my transformation.

The hardest thing I had to do after the skydiving tunnel accident on June 3, 2019, was make the twenty-five-mile drive home that night using only my right hand and arm. I tried to drive with my left, but there was intense pain, and I had absolutely no control of the wheel. It might have been the longest, most painful drive I had ever made, fearful that my right arm and hand would fail me and cause an auto accident, on top of whatever the heck was going on with my left shoulder. Between the pain and worry, I was a nervous wreck. I had to totally depend on my right side—the thought of engaging in daily activities, including typing this very manuscript, seemed overwhelming and impossible.

I am extremely grateful for the eight years of preparation that came before this difficult moment. Without my transformation, I doubt I would have had the passion, drive, and persistence to handle it. Neurologically speaking, it seems to have paid dividends. For if this had happened before my transformation in 2011, I wouldn't have been able to function at all. I would have been utterly dependent on others.

In the book *The Boy Who Could Run but Not Walk*, Dr. Karen Pape talks about her proven protocol in young kids. The act of restraining their dominant side ensures that they will use their nondominant cerebral palsy side and develop neural pathways, pathways that could not have developed if their dominant side were allowed to take over. This is known as constraint-induced movement therapy (CI or CIMT) and is used to increase the use of an affected limb as the result of CP, stroke, or other brain injury. Dr. Pape adds that CIMT aims at decreasing the effects of learned nonuse.[61] Unfortunately, CIMT is more commonly used in adults recovering from a stroke than in children or adults like me with similar types of brain injury or CP. In my case, I had been in a left-arm immobilizer sling for 196 very long days (twenty-eight weeks), having to rely solely on my right side to do everything.[62] Now, isn't that a case for Dr. Pape's study? Only, in my case, it was fifty years post–kid stage of life. Bottom line, I was pretty impressed with what I was able to achieve every day by utilizing just my right side while in that imprisoning sling. Improvements and new achievements came every day, faster than I could fully comprehend or even keep track of.

DRIVING CHALLENGES

Remember my old Datsun stick shift? Fast-forward to June 2019: I had been using my left hand to steer my car up to this pivotal point of time, and now that I had an automatic transmission, my right hand and left foot no longer had to work for a paycheck, until now. Due to my multiple left arm and shoulder surgeries, I had to take what I was learning in the gym and apply it to driving. It was time to accelerate the process, to build *stronger* neural pathways and alter brain muscle maps. At first, it was extremely tough knowing what to do, and when…and having confidence in my ability to perform under the stress of driving, especially on the roads in Austin. It was fascinating to see this transformation in real time. I was directly experiencing Dr. Karen Pape's restraint theory in action. Now that my left arm was in a sling and I no longer had a safety net to fall back on, I had to become really good at driving right-handed and even putting on my seatbelt and fastening that little thin buckle into its receiver on the first attempt.[63] Never had I thought about how much dexterity fastening a *simple* seatbelt actually required. Today it almost feels like a natural movement. This was further proof of new neural-pathway development becoming second nature in me.

THE LONG ROAD TO RECOVERY

Following my skydiving accident and multiple surgeries, I began to count the days and weeks in reference to post–shoulder surgery number two, which occurred on August 1, 2019. Just like shoulder surgery number one, I spent weeks one and two mostly incoherent and in lots of pain, immobilized and on strong painkillers, intravenous regional anesthesia, intravenous catheter nerve blocks, and other medications. I do not remember much from this time period. However, I do remember wearing a high-tech radiator-type cooling sleeve on my left shoulder and chest area that allowed ice water to circulate through connected pipes of the sleeve to keep my swelling and inflammation at bay for about a month or so.[64] I had to keep refilling the water container with ice every four to six hours. That was my official timekeeping method during this period. When the water ceased to be cold, the pain increased, and I would again need help refilling the ice for another four to six hours. This ran on twenty-four hours a day.

After week number three, my intravenous (IV) nerve block had run its course, and I was able to remove the IV catheter that was positioned on the nerve root in my neck—ouch. By this point (after three surgeries and three nerve blocks), I was a master at having these IVs removed from my neck. My first postoperative checkup was good—all going per my doctor's plan. I was allowed and encouraged to cautiously step back into the gym. And although I would do it, this was something I no longer had any interest in doing. After all, I had gone through this twice before with both my biceps and first shoulder rehabilitation protocols. I was up to bat for a third time, and a strikeout was foremost on my mind. I was heading into flight mode fast. Not again. I did not want to be in a gym and only allowed to perform nonimpact cardio.

So, what the hell am I doing? What is the use in being here? After all, I was once able to do everything in here, and now, again, I am limited to only a recumbent bike. Why even bother?

My thoughts were back. Just like in the beginning, nine years ago, as well as just a few weeks back, this place was once again far outside my limited reach. Not only did I have CP, but now my non-CP side was immobile. My balance was off once again, and I was limited in what I could do. Moreover, I was starting to gain weight. I learned later that it was known as *post-operation weight gain* due to multiple factors, like (1) the stress of the injury and surgeries (trauma) inflicted on the body, (2) various medications and painkillers that can trigger metabolic system changes and hormonal imbalances, and (3) rest and recovery changes, as rest will slow down the body's basal metabolic rate, which can all lead to weight gain.

This all took place within a very short time frame, and with three surgeries under my belt, I was ripe for this weight gain. It was also apparent that my hormones were messed up, as my blood work looked like Dr. Leonard McCoy from *Star Trek* needed to do a complete medical examination of me aboard the starship *Enterprise*.

I have learned over many years of training that maintaining a routine is particularly important, from both a psychological and physiological standpoint. Varying a routine is wise and warranted, but it's a routine nonetheless. It was time for me to start praying for strength and clawing my way back up the recovery ladder once again, for the third time, getting back to the basics, even if I no longer had a trainer by my side.

"Cerebral palsy should not keep one from reaching the impossible" was something that I had said a lot during those early years. Now it was time for me to start believing, once more, in what I had said so often before. I also kept repeating Philippians 4:13, "I can do all things through Christ who gives me strength." That verse and a drive deep within me were once again winning me over and reminding me *now* that it was time for me to begin my recovery in a new light, *His* light. Let the slow and painful process of strengthening once more be for His glory and part of His process in the aftermath of my reckoning.

By week eight, I had post-op checkup number two. I was relieved that I had made it one week longer than the last surgery, and I was hoping for some good news (unlike last time). Fortunately, per doctor's orders, I was finally able to remove the splint from my left arm outside of therapy for very, very short periods of time. It would allow for a bit of fresh air, especially around the house or while I was sitting at work. I must admit, I did not want to remove or replace my splint. It was painful and difficult to do with my right hand, and trying to get my left arm to fully extend and move around was nearly impossible at first. *Houston, we have a left-arm system failure here*, I kept thinking to myself. I could not believe how much my left arm had atrophied in twenty-eight weeks (196 days). However, I did feel some freedom from the bondage at last, even if it was only for minutes at a time.

The next couple of weeks, during my outpatient rehab sessions at Symmetry Physical Therapy of Austin, I experienced painful but glorious freedom outside of my splint as Brad Bevil, my physical therapist, performed simple ROM and passive movement exercises. Due to the extent of my injuries and the complexity of my surgeries, Brad took it slow and easy. I experienced lots of tingling in my arm and hand, but everything was looking good. The X-rays and sonograms showed that the healing was progressing as expected.

By week ten, I was somewhat free from my splint, except in crowds and unfamiliar places where I might be tempted to use my arm to lift or move objects that could cause damage to my shoulder. I had to be incredibly careful. I continued to experience intense tingling in my left hand and lower arm— sort of like when your hand falls asleep and you try to move it, like pins and needles. The doctor and PT staff said that this would lessen in time. I had my doubts, but I was hopeful. The tingling lasted for several months.

AN UNEXPECTED GIFT—MY ADOPTION, REVISITED

As I mentioned earlier, after all my shoulder surgeries, I was pretty banged up. I was in an arm sling, looked like a hot mess, and was only allowed to use one piece of equipment in the entire gym: my old friend, the Octane Fitness lateral slide machine. Well, my doctor preferred that I stick to a recumbent bike. However, it was not all about the bike. I knew I could do more. Here enters Lauren Wolf into my life, marching right up to the same machine as me to do a quick cardio workout and leave. What seemed to be a "random" encounter ended up changing the course of not only my life and hers, but countless others to come (spoiler alert).

To say Lauren stayed active is quite an understatement. With three young kids under seven, a loving husband, and an extensive workload, she had very little free time. Her hectic work and home schedule for this particular day only allowed her a limited workout, so she was determined to get through her cardio session and return home before her kids awoke from naptime.

Today, we both enjoy embellishing this story by adding in little bits of fiction, like that she saw me in a splint, all tattered, beat me up, and kicked me to the floor, just to get her cardio completed in time. Comical as it sounds, at that point in my recovery, it would have only taken a slight finger tap from her, and I would have been down for the count.

We ended up performing our cardio sessions side by side on identical machines once the other machine next to mine became free. Some courteous small talk piqued her investigative spirit. As it turned out, Lauren had worked for Pulitzer Prize–winning writer Lawrence Wright as a fact checker and research assistant for his book *Going Clear: Scientology, Hollywood, and the Prison of Belief*. She had also served as an associate producer on HBO's Emmy Award–winning documentary *Going Clear*.

As she learned of my ongoing transformation and this very book project, she grew interested in learning more. After further conversation, she realized the nature of my cerebral palsy was similar to someone she knew well. My story became personal to her, and she was even more intrigued. Upon further interviewing, she also learned of my adoption and not knowing where I came from. I had unknowingly hooked my first investigative journalist! She was all in. Lauren's passion for genealogy and her investigative nature ultimately led her to come alongside me and add a brand-new dimension to my transformation that I never would have explored if not for this encounter—of my genealogy and birth family.

Lauren now had a new story to uncover…me! She proceeded to tell me of her passion for helping adopted *kids* reunite with their birth families. She asked if I was interested. I think I said something like "Hell, yes!"

As we talked and got to know each other, she explained that she wanted to investigate my adoption and genetic heritage. I was hooked on every word she had to say. From an early age, my parents had told me that I was adopted. I was grateful to know this from the beginning of my childhood. I knew my adoptive family loved me, so there was never any ill will toward them or my biological family. I had always been curious but never knew just how to go about exploring my heritage, and I did not want to go through this alone. Up to now, I had not possessed the "key" to unlocking this door. What lay beyond it were answers to questions such as *Do I have any other siblings out there?* and *Does anyone from my birth family even know I exist?*

As I began writing this book, these questions perplexed me even more. When Lauren and I met, she became the key to unlocking this adoption door.

As we continued talking, she educated me about the various advancements in family mapping using DNA and that it was now possible to find out where I came from. A simple DNA test, and locating my biological family was not only possible but easy (for her, perhaps) through a process she had successfully employed before with others. All I needed to do was set up an account on Ancestry.com and order a DNA test kit. I could not order a test kit fast enough. After what seemed like an eternity, my results were in, and Lauren went to work uncovering my past.

Armed with my DNA results and her expert investigative techniques, her research uncovered a mountain of information about me, such as the facts that I came from a large family of Swedish and German heritage and that my birth family was now mostly located in Oregon. Lauren also discovered that I look strikingly similar to a photo she found of my maternal grandfather. In fact, dress me up like my grandfather and take an old-time photo, and I could easily pass as his double.

Seeing this comparison was how I knew Lauren and I were on the right path.

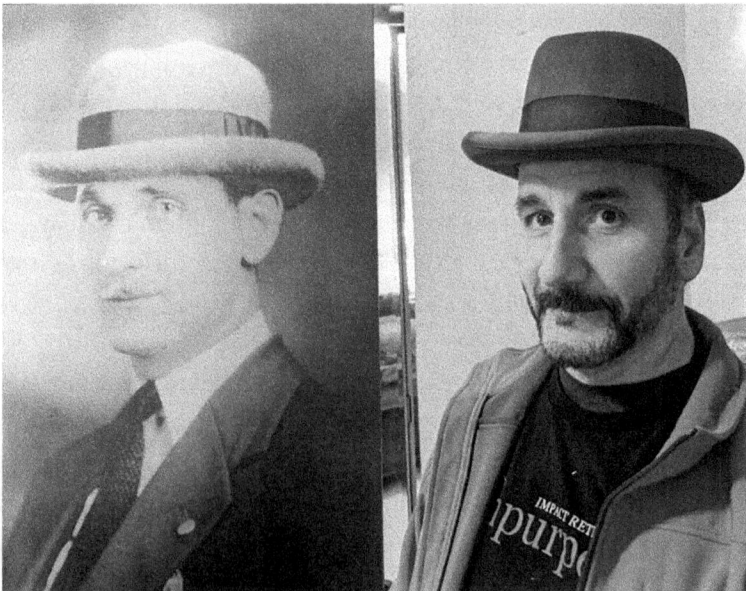

Picture of my grandfather (left) next to a picture of me (right)

Lauren discovered that on my birth mother's side of my family, I had a single half-brother, and on my birth father's side, I had three half-sisters and two half-brothers, as well as more cousins on both sides than I could keep track of at this point. My birth father had passed away in 2002, but my birth mother was currently living in Oregon. Lauren created a very professional "first contact letter." She sent the photo of my maternal grandfather and a photo of me to my birth mother, and we waited patiently for a reply. Was I going to get to meet my birth mother after more than fifty years?

Lauren also discovered that there was no cancer or genetic concerns anywhere in my family line. It seemed that my genetic makeup was strong and healthy. Knowing this medical history was a huge relief in itself, as I had always wondered about what I would face growing older.

After a couple of months with no reply, Lauren's plan was to make "first contact" with one of my cousins, then my half-siblings. As it turned out, one of my siblings had already noticed the addition of me in their family tree on Ancestry.com and was curious to know more. They say nothing travels faster than the speed of light—except gossip. Well, the news of me spread around *the family* like wildfire. I started to get inquiries from everywhere. My various calls and visits were all fantastic, and my fear about meeting my long-lost biological family was put more at ease with every conversation. To my great surprise, everyone Lauren contacted or who contacted us was eager to know more about where I had come from, and they could not wait to meet their long-lost relative. Meeting my various biological family members was incredible. Learning about my genetic family and traits was like opening a chest filled with priceless treasure. The most emotional call I made was to my half-bother on my mother's side. He had grown up as an only child, until now. Upon meeting, I learned that my birth mother had suffered a major stroke around the same time Lauren had sent the letter to her. As I write this, we don't know if she saw the letter before she was hospitalized, as my brother never located the letter. Time will tell if I will be able to meet my birth mother.

I am now in the process of connecting with my extended biological family and learning more about my heritage every day.

By meeting Lauren in that gym while in a broken and beaten-down condition, I was further led along an unexpected path in my transformation, transforming not who I had become but where I had come from. Every day brings news from the biological side of my family, and it is a real joy to keep uncovering new facets to my heritage as I continue to heal and rehab.

THE HEALING HAD JUST BEGUN

As I mentioned earlier, one of the hardest and most unexpected struggles of fighting multiple uphill battles over a long rehabilitation regimen is *trust*. When professionals have failed you—by walking away or by outright causing an injury—having trust in professionals becomes exceedingly difficult moving forward.

By this point of my recovery, it had been over a year and a half since hitting the wall and incurring shoulder damage, and I was still in constant pain. Rehab and PT continued, and I often had the sense that I would never fully recover from this nightmare. To top that off, the question of how to deal with trusting any professional was at the forefront of my mind as I forged slowly ahead on my long road called recovery. As I mentioned earlier, leaning on my own understanding would no longer suffice. I had to let Him steer the ship through this ongoing reckoning. Over time, with a lot of prayer and lots of deep soul-searching, I would be led to a new team that would soon come alongside me in my transformation. The healing had truly just begun.

PART 10

Transformation through Neuroplasticity

The Ultimate Change Engine

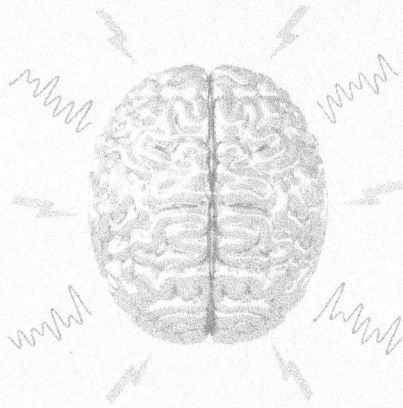

Scott's Transformation Alliances Begin

RADICAL LEAPS FORWARD OFTEN HAPPEN WHEN WE LEAST EXPECT them. Even before *the reckoning*, when I was still on top of my "A game" and training three days a week with Ruth (early 2018), I had started researching several technologies that would further enhance my brain–muscle alliance. The scientist and engineer in me wanted to perform a deep dive in understanding how Mighty Mouse was able to fly and just how high he could go. In the back of my mind, I wondered if Mighty Mouse could actually skydive again. Ultimately, I wanted to share my research and replicate what I had learned with others so that you, my readers, would benefit in your own transformations. I began researching the latest technologies for helping prime the brain and muscles to perform better and faster (cue the music from *The Six Million Dollar Man*). I had spent a great amount of time learning and partnering with several of these technologies, even integrating some of them into my prior workout sessions with Ruth.

Two modalities especially held my interest. These were neural priming and electrical muscle stimulation. Neural priming of the brain is like the "ready, set" before the "go" prior to an activity. The theory is that priming muscles increases their initial speed of response, giving us the added edge when time of response is critical, as in the fight-or-flight response (sympathetic nervous system). Priming of muscles and other senses alerts the brain to get ready for more input. In theory, neural priming can increase attention, focus, readiness, and accuracy of the body's responses to stimuli. During year three of my transformation, while I was still training with Ruth in 2015, Halo Neuroscience and I partnered to study their Halo Sport headsets for people with CP. The Halo Sport headsets are designed to increase the brain's neuroplasticity, so you can create and strengthen motor pathways faster. They call this hyper-plasticity, or hyper-learning.[65]

Their headset worked by applying a small electric current to the part of the brain that controls movement, activating neurons so they would fire more often when you train. The more neurons that fired together, the faster pathways were built in the brain.

I worked with these folks and the Halo Sport for about a year before my study ended, and I stopped using their product when the headset they provided had issues. Although this technology could be very promising for folks with CP and stroke, Ruth and I were not able to forge forward with testing their product due to lack of support.

However, the modality of electrical muscle stimulation seemed to show great promise and hold a bright future in my transformation. Called electrical muscle stimulation, or ESTIM for short, this technology sparked my interest from my initial research with Dr. Karen Pape's intensive work with people with CP.

In Dr. Pape's book, she talks about utilizing Russian stimulation, or neuro-muscular electrical stimulation (NMES) to build muscle mass in Michelle, a young girl living in an acute care hospital with no expectations of ever leaving.[66] This was a brand-new concept, and not all therapists were using it. The theory Dr. Pape proposed was that during the initial period of immobility, Michelle's muscles got weaker and weaker. As her spinal shock resolved and she tried to move, she lacked the strength to do it. Her muscles were not strong enough to move her against the force of gravity.

Electrical stimulation was a technology that had been shown to help strengthen weak and underutilized muscles. It worked for adults. It was reasonable to think that it would work for children like Michelle as well. Dr. Pape utilized low-intensity NMES for longer periods of time than her earlier traditional high-intensity Russian stimulation, and the results were simply astounding. After about five weeks of electrical stimulation, Michelle was on the mat, and she pushed herself up into the sitting position and said, "Look! Look at me! Look what I've done!"[67] Within six months, she was able to crawl, control her bladder, and be taken off the ventilator for long periods of time. After eight months, she was up and walking with a walker. She eventually moved home for high school. Dr. Pape gave this treatment the initial name therapeutic electrical stimulation (TES).[68] She went on to use TES on her patients with cerebral palsy. All the children with CP who completed her study showed great positive change.[69]

In Dr. Karen Pape's book, she tells us of a January 1993 *Canadian Medical Association Journal* article that was written by a freelance writer, Olga Lachky, who gave a positive account of Pape's work.[70] The writer picked up on the underlying argument about neuroplasticity. "By wedding the laboratory concept of neuroplasticity—the apparent ability of the brain either to repair damaged areas over time or to find alternative pathways around an injury—to new home-based technologies that stimulate and repair mechanisms," Olga concludes, "Pape and her colleagues have offered new hope to more than 2,000 patients since the Magee Clinic opened its doors in 1989."[71]

The desire to dig deeper into this therapeutic technology called ESTIM was now extraordinarily strong in me, and it seemed the perfect time to invest. Now was the time to "amp up Mighty Mouse."[72]

ESTIM—MY TRANSFORMATION

On September 10, 2019, seven weeks after shoulder surgery number two, I took the electrical leap into ESTIM full throttle. Enter Garrett Salpeter, known as "The Health Engineer." Garrett used his education in engineering neuroscience to create NeuFit, short for NEUrological FITness. He first learned about the paramount importance of the nervous system when dealing with an injury of his own. As an ice hockey player, he tore some ligaments and was supposed to have surgery and be out for over three months. He figured this would be the case, as it seemed in line with his previous experiences in the traditional physical therapy and orthopedic realms.

Serendipitously, Garrett met a chiropractic neurologist who introduced him to functional neurology and primitive forms of monophasic direct-current ESTIM. By taking a functional approach to a problem that was typically thought of as being purely structural, he was able to heal his ligaments in three weeks and avoid surgery altogether. This neurological approach worked so well that he never looked back.

Garrett was inspired to share the healing potential of this neurological approach to treatment after he experienced its effects firsthand. But even as he continued to witness the therapeutic impacts of the neurology-first approach—and learn more about electrical current's power to reeducate the nervous system—he realized there was a missing piece.[73]

Like me, Garrett became determined to learn as much as possible about how to work with the nervous system. To that end, he spent hundreds of hours in self-study, mentored under several leading-edge practitioners, and tested many of his theories on himself and others. He even went back to school for a PhD program in neuroscience, a program that he eventually left so he could launch a company and invent the Neubie device based on monophasic pulse technology, with several added bonuses in the mix.

In 2009, he opened his first facility in Austin, Texas, to start sharing his Neubie device and methods within the community. This has grown into what is now known as NeuFit, which combines an advanced understanding of physiology with the best practices from diverse training and therapeutic practices and constantly pushes these processes by using technology to accelerate them further. Since that first day, he has worked with people of all ages and in almost all situations, including athletes from MLB, the NFL, the NHL, the NBA, UFC, the Olympics, and the NCAA, and people recovering from stroke, spinal cord injury, and multiple sclerosis—and soon to add CP to this list. He has certified hundreds of practitioners in the NeuFit Method and is humbled at seeing those practitioners "pay it forward" by helping hundreds of thousands of people live life at a higher level by eliminating pain, improving performance, and even sometimes avoiding surgeries altogether.

I wanted to meet and come alongside Garrett and see if his NeuFit program could work for people like me, with the added bonus of speeding up rehab from multiple left-arm and shoulder surgeries. My transformation and post-surgery case seemed extraordinarily complex. However, it was not too far removed from his work and his life story.

It took me a few weeks to get up the nerve to call and set up a meeting with Garrett. After all, I was in a brace and must have looked like Dean Winters as "Mayhem" from those Allstate commercials. I hardly looked like an athlete undergoing a transformation by this time. Showing up to a meeting wearing a shoulder brace, sporting a weakened body with CP and a beard to match, I must have looked like a cross between John Wick and Mayhem—not a promising sight for sure. I even had the bandages and props to boot. To say that I was nervous about this meeting was an understatement. Besides, I was a little unsure if this technology he had developed would work for me and other people with CP, or if he would take me seriously at all. However, as soon as we met, Garrett's calm, warm, intelligent personality put me at ease about any concern I may have felt. He did not see me as "broken" or weak. He saw me as a determined athlete, engineer, and researcher like him, ready to prove my theory. Mighty Mouse was ready for a new cape and maze.

Garrett and I met at his West Austin headquarters, where he showed me his Neubie system and recommended that I read the book *The Brain That Changes Itself* by Dr. Norman Doidge. This book gave numerous examples of neuroplasticity, and it fit right in with Dr. Karen Pape's work, which I had been studying for so long. As it turned out, Dr. Doidge had written the preface to Dr. Pape's book. I read Dr. Doidge's book before and after my left-shoulder rehab session each day and wanted to experience this amazing transformation for myself.

During our various visits, I shared with Garrett my life journey with CP: my transformation story, my triumphs and various gains, and hitting the wall that led me to our visit. I even shared a very early version of my book manuscript. Garrett then let me in on his latest book project, entitled *The NeuFit Method: Unleash the Power of the Nervous System for Faster Healing and Optimal Performance* (now available). One chapter is even on neuroplasticity for a range of neurological diagnoses like CP, stroke, spinal cord injury, and even multiple sclerosis. Garrett introduced me to his staff and gave me the dollar tour. It was an impressive place nestled in West Lake Hills, off Capital of Texas Highway (a.k.a. Loop 360), near a well-known barbecue place that I had frequented many times before. A small gym-style workout floor was located on the main level, complete with seven identical workout bays with weights and Neubies at each station. His facility included two physical therapy rooms for individual PT/OT work and a large room upstairs for group-style classes.

Garrett was intrigued with my transformation progress over the prior eight years, along with what had happened recently to my left shoulder. After all, it was a little hard to hide a splinted arm. He was also intrigued by my CP research and the vision I had in mind. He thought that his NeuFit methodology could be greatly beneficial for both my right CP side as well as rehabilitating my left side once it had sufficiently healed and was ready for this stage of rehab.

First, he said we must correct those "maladaptive habits and movements" that had been established early in my life. I explained to him that in my research, I had come up with the analogy that the motor nervous system in our body is like driving on a road. Muscle memory had been created to move and function. However, certain movements were maladaptive due to early years with

CP, before my brain had healed, around age two. I then told him that this was similar to my "pothole in the road" analogy (mentioned earlier). Garrett agreed with this analogy and said we had to retrain my brain to efficiently and effortlessly drive straight over where that pothole used to be (build new neural pathways). This is the basis of neuroplasticity and what NeuFit could help me achieve—to learn to drive my muscle-memory "circuits" correctly. Dr. Karen Pape described it like this: "Habits are not broken or changed; they are replaced."[74]

Goal-oriented therapy was the way I had been proceeding over these past few years, recording everything, including goals and corresponding results. I now needed Garrett's help to push forward through the next phase—I needed clear, measurable goals and metrics to see if the effects of his Neubie would really pay off. He knew that it would. Garrett went on to explain that the Neubie is short for "NEUro-Bio-Electric Stimulator." When the Neubie is combined with the NeuFit Method, this synergy provides protocols for neuromuscular reeducation.[75] The nervous system controls every muscle movement. Like a garden hose, sometimes the nervous system gets a "kink" in it. The Neubie helps in "unkinking" the hose and reeducating these pathways to function properly. He was sure that this would benefit me in both the right and left sides of my body.

I was so excited about his ideas for my treatment that I could hardly wait to begin.

Garrett soon introduced me to a member of his staff, Ed Patterson. Ed would become my physical therapist for a custom program designed to stimulate and correct my right-side neural pathways and rehab the left side of my body with the Neubie.

Ed started working with my right side first as my left shoulder rehab progressed at Symmetry PT, and when my left arm was ready, Ed introduced the NeuFit Method to my whole body. Our early work consisted of slow, deep nose breathing while performing a "master resetting,"[76] which is a technique to increase function in my vagus nerve[77] and activate my parasympathetic nervous system.[78] Then we progressed into right-side therapy, which included dexterity and strengthening protocols. Starting with my fingers and hand dexterity, I learned how to properly strengthen my wrist and how to turn my wrist to the right and left (radial deviation to ulnar deviation), then we worked on flexion and extension of my arm (bending and straightening). Ed also conducted legwork, working on balance and proper foot alignment, and my toes as well. By incorporating Dr. Pape's theories, the Neubie, and the NeuFit Method into a custom plan, I began to strengthen my "partner muscles" and develop stronger neural circuits to keep my "bully muscles" from taking over. This allowed for elegance in movement on my right side.

Waking up pathways and building stronger neural networks on my right side in Ed's therapy room was simply amazing. My body was learning exciting new stuff like never before. I would reinforce these movements and exercises immediately afterwards in a gym setting. Repetitively and systematically energizing these new pathways and "building new roads" within my body (nervous system) was indeed working. In fact, it worked like lighter fluid on a flame. It magnified changes in my brain muscle maps at an even more accelerated pace than before the reckoning. Plug me in…time to amp it up and become the energizer mouse.

Athletes will practice specific movements over and over again, and I was no different. But I would soon realize that "practice does not make perfect," as Vince Lombardi once said. "Only perfect practice makes perfect." If you practice a movement incorrectly, this practice can lead to maladaptive muscle maps, as stated earlier by Dr. Karen Pape. Only in performing muscle patterns perfectly every time does this become efficient and *perfect* in execution. Adding pulsed galvanic monophasic ESTIM into this perfect practice accelerated new muscle-memory response in my body even further. It seemed that Garrett's Neubie and NeuFit Method were the answer to building the new and lasting pathways that I had been searching for.

TIME ACCELERATES

By September 2019, I was in rehabilitation physical therapy three days a week at Symmetry for my left shoulder and neural therapy on my right side for two days a week at NeuFit, for a total of five days every week. I wanted to maximize my recovery by working on my right-side CP neurological strengthening and increasing range of active motion while working on my left-side rehab at the same time. My various doctors were still somewhat pessimistic about what NeuFit electrical stimulation could accomplish. I'd had CP my entire life, they said. They didn't think it would help. However, my general practitioner was on board and said he would help in any way he could.

By week twenty-four (on January 15, 2020), six long months from my shoulder revision surgery and over a year after my biceps surgery, I received some exceptionally good and unexpected news from Dr. Hall. After more X-rays, sonograms, reviews of my physical therapist's reports, and a thorough evaluation, Dr. Hall recommended I progress to the next stage of recovery: weight-bearing PT via professional certified trainer. He recommended that I continue moving aggressively into this phase of recovery with a highly skilled and trusted trainer—someone like Ruth. Still leery of ever hiring a personal trainer ever again, I told him I would take it under advisement.

There would be no more functional physical therapy on my left side. It was now time for me to get up enough nerve to find a new personal trainer whom I could trust and start weight-bearing and strengthening work, rebuilding my left side along with my "new and improved" right side as an athlete and bodybuilder. The crazy thing was that my right side was now stronger than my left side. This was a complete role reversal from when I started personal training over nine years ago and was, with good reason, mind-blowing to me and many others. I just wish I could have celebrated this news with the trainer who had begun this awesome transformation nine years back.

A NEW BEGINNING

December 30, 2019, was my last session with Brad, my physical therapist over at Symmetry. I was cleared to begin weight-bearing loading on my left side. Since I was highly encouraged by both Dr. Hall and Brad to return to personal training with a certified trainer, I started my search. Phase four of my rehab was about to begin. But who would be up for the challenge? Who could I trust? Who had the skillset to safely bring me to this new level? I needed someone who truly knew what I could achieve—someone who would come alongside me, encourage this broken spirit, and safely build me back up and beyond from these many setbacks—I needed a true professional. This was going to be an incredibly challenging "ask."

FINDING A NEW TRIGGER—THE LACROSSE BALL BOUNCE TECHNIQUE

I found that running laps was now impossible due to both psychological and physiological reasons. Now that my trainer had left, the concept of "take a lap" no longer had the same psychological effect as before. Anyone who has ever been in the military could tell you that no one has ever been motivated by giving themselves a lap. Physiologically, I was unable to run due to the jarring motion on my left shoulder, a move that was strictly off limits for now. So I had to find a new trigger to get my brain to disengage from the "can't-do" attitude and engage in the "can-do" attitude.

The brain loves novelty; it wires new pathways faster when utilizing novelty in learning. I found that bouncing a lacrosse ball from my left hand to my right hand, firmly catching it, then bouncing it back to my left hand, catching it, and repeating this cycle for several minutes was effective physical therapy for my left shoulder while also energizing my corpus callosum, those two hundred million axons cross-wiring circuits that exist in our brains that connect our right and left hemispheres. I was building new and stronger pathways deep within my brain, with the added benefit of building brand-new muscle memory for my right-hand coordination and dexterity for reach, grab, hold, then throw back, along with eye-hand coordination. This was just the novelty that my brain needed to not only perform whatever task I should be doing correctly but also to get me out of my own head.

To ratchet this novelty up a notch or two, I superset this into both my physical therapy routine and my workouts. Notch two was to integrate this technique (left-right lacrosse ball bounce) while standing on a BOSU ball or while walking down the hall. Up until six months before the reckoning, I was not able to catch a ball at all right-handed. Now I am walking down the hall bouncing a ball from one hand to the other, as well as on an unstable platform. That is true neuroplasticity in action! My next notch (number three) was mastering the bouncing of a lacrosse ball while balancing on my knees on a stability ball. Mighty mouse was apparently interviewing for the circus.

RECONCILIATION AND GIVING GRACE

A long-term professional relationship with a personal trainer often becomes a very close friendship, and it can be difficult when the relationship ends. A good trainer is one who coaches, inspires, and motivates, one who sees and conveys potential in you (the trainee)—and it's their job to help instill this positive attitude into you, at least if they're good at their job. I mentioned previously that there's a "building up," both psychologically and physiologically, that occurs here—that's what a good trainer does. There's the element of money, of course, but there's still a genuine concern for your well-being, especially over many years. Your trainer shares in your triumphs and achievements as well as the pain that you must endure for gains to occur. This is what had transpired over the prior eight years of my athletic life with Ruth.

Going back and trying to reconcile this relationship with Ruth seemed pointless from most of my friends' and family's point of view. My closest friends kept telling me that Ruth did nothing but abandon me during my greatest time of need. However, I thought it was important to try to mend the bruised and battered relationship between us, even if we never trained together again. Up to this point, showing grace was something that I was not particularly good at, and God was telling me over and over that I needed to provide ample grace and forgiveness to my former trainer.

Where to start reconciling was foremost in my thoughts. Ruth had never been a good communicator, even while we were training together, which would make this even harder. Reconciling even made it into my dreams. How messed up was that? I had to attempt to resolve this before I went insane or drove my friends insane while I was processing all of this. Ruth had very seldom acknowledged or replied to my texts and calls, even during the best of times. Now it was like a broadcast when I would reach out. My messages were always transmitted, but were they ever received? Whoever listens to broadcasts anyway? Just a lot of dead air for most of us.

On January 16, 2020, I decided to make a visit to my former gym, where Ruth worked as the fitness manager and where so many of our past "wins" had occurred. It was awfully hard to walk in that door. I actually sat in my car for fifteen minutes, psyching myself up. Upon entering, seeing my picture still up on the counter as a 2019 Gold's transformation challenge club winner filled me with even more anxiety. The voices were back. *What in the heck are you doing in here, Scott?* I felt so uncomfortable and way out of place.

I made a beeline to the dressing room, changed, and started on the routine I'd so often employed in the past. *Stay focused*, I kept thinking. I had my headphones on my head, but I never actually hit *play* on my iPhone. I wanted to observe my surroundings. I kept a lookout for Ruth, all senses on high alert, ready to bolt at any moment (flight response trying to reassert itself). Warm-up completed? Check. *Now what?* Oh yes! The Smith bar machine was open. *Perfect*, I thought. I quickly headed over to claim my spot. Setting up for some on-the-ground, single right-arm chest presses would be a good way to try out my doctor's orders, I figured. While I was loading up my weights onto the bar and descending into position on my back on the floor, there was Ruth, approaching me.

Hold it together, Scott, I heard in my head. *Breathe! Keep it positive and upbeat.* After all, I was no longer under her training. I was a free agent. Why was I scared that I was doing something wrong already? *Snap out of it! Smile and say "Hi,"* the voice in my head commanded.

Before I could stand up, I heard Ruth say, "Hey, what are you doing?" as if nothing was wrong.

"Doing a little pressing from ground level," I replied cautiously. "Like in the old days."

More small talk followed, but I was unable to really hear or comprehend any of it due to my fast-beating heart in my ears. I apologized for anything I may have done. I said that I was frustrated and angry and unable to fully process and convey what had happened with my skydiving accident and the fallout between us (not wanting to bring up the ghosting point of view). By this point, I felt extremely nervous, timid like the little mouse from the old days. I held a firm stance.

"That's okay," she said. "The videos and photos from what we were doing for the book can be saved for later," she added, changing the subject.

What's okay? I wondered. *And why would she bring up videos of my training at a time like this?*

Her comments struck me as rather odd, since she had walked away from me and given the implicit impression that she wanted nothing to do with me after the accident. Why would she save videos and photos if she wanted nothing to do with me? My mind started to spin again. But I decided to drop this line of thinking and forge ahead.

Before I knew it, she asked what I was doing the following week. I said I had that next Monday off because of the Martin Luther King Jr. holiday (January 20, 2020). She suggested we get together for measurements. "Let's schedule a time to come in." She said to call, and we would set up a time. It all felt strange but promising.

That evening's one-hour drive home was difficult. Processing what had just happened took a great deal of brainpower, and my feelings were all over the map. Were we even in the same rulebook or playing the same sport here? It made no sense. But I've seen stranger things, so I was going with it to see what developed.

The next day, I sent a text and a voicemail to schedule a time to meet. No response. Two days went by, three, then five. Communications had once again failed. MLK day came and went. This was simply crazy.

One week later, I once again showed up at her gym. I was on an elliptical trainer when she spotted me and approached. Again, this seemed odd since she was not in the habit of finding clients, or ex-clients, out on the workout floor. Ruth and I had a very brief talk, if you could even call it that. She was visibly upset and seemed emotional. She had trouble making direct eye contact with me, and she did not say much. It felt like something was keeping her from reaching out, from being able to help repair this trainer–trainee relationship. Some unspoken influence. Her few words cut through me like a hot knife through butter.

When I told her that my doctor wanted me to start working with a trainer again, she said, "Just look at one of our old training cards; you know what to do." I was perplexed. My heart sank as I realized what she meant—she was not interested in working with me any longer.

No explanation, no reason given, and just like that, on January 24, 2020, after eight years of training, it became official: I had lost an incredibly good friend, my advocate, and my mentor. She had been instrumental in kicking off this transformation after my first session with her way back in 2011. It appeared she had to work out what was going on in her own head, but for me, I had given my all, and still it seemed not enough.

It was time for the next chapter to begin. I decided to pick up what was left of my shattered spirit and never return to her gym again. Time to move on to a new phase of training—a new season. I felt like I had done all I could do. It was time to move forward. My conscience was now clean, and I no longer had dreams of this dilemma again.

PART 11

A New Day

With Him Nothing Is Impossible

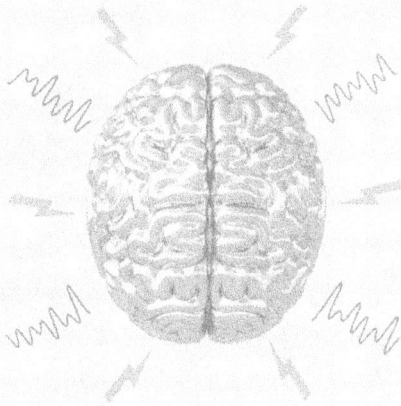

A New Beginning— the Reunion

I SAT AT HOME, PRAYING, "WHO SHALL I FIND AS A NEW TRAINER THAT I can trust to safely push me farther than I think I can go?" And on February 3, 2020, my prayers were answered.

I had narrowed my list down to a small number of potentials I had researched, met with, and interviewed, but none had earned my final approval for one reason or another—after all, I had high standards. I prayed and I listened. I heard a small voice whisper, *Text Brian Williams and say hello*. Brian was my trainer when I received the "Train or Die" hooded sweatshirt from that other bodybuilder, and I could not get that hoodie out of my head.[79] I sensed that Brian would be my next trainer. I texted and asked if he was still training and if he was interested in training me again after all this time. To my surprise, he responded to my text right away and asked, "What about your current trainer, Ruth?"

"Very long story," was my reply.

"Sure. Let's meet up at my new gym and talk," he said.

It seemed perfect that Brian and I would train again. Not only did Brian know me and my abilities, but he also understood complex injuries that athletes like me often endure. He believed in my potential and knew of my CP. I knew his training style and trusted him to push me forward.

Today was a new day, a new gym, and a new stage in my training life. Brian was excited that I wanted to train with him again. We were both eager to pick up where we'd left off, with a few new challenges added to the mix. I was ready to "get froggy" once again, a term Brian had often used back in 2017. I think it was his way of saying *let's hop to it.*

MIGHTY MOUSE RETURNS TO BODYBUILDING

I had my first workout with Brian at his new gym on February 3, 2020, and it was awesome. He was now at Crunch Fitness, a club not far from the location where we had once trained up in Round Rock, Texas. He introduced me to his staff, showed me around, and wanted to see what I could do at this stage of rehab. During our first session, he even commented that my right hand had never gripped and lifted as much weight as he was now seeing me lift. He went on to say that I could not do this back in the "old days." I had just lifted a fifty-pound kettlebell right-handed while balancing on a tractor tire. Grip and form on my right side were now far superior to what he had known before, and far greater than my left could currently do. I was pumped, to say the least. He said that I was ready to bring my left side up to where my CP right side was performing. Who would have thought? A concept 180 degrees from my pre-reckoning days. My new brain muscle map had changed so much that my conscious mind had a hard time believing it. I knew that I was indeed alive and about to begin a whole new transformation.

God lovingly pushes His children to do the impossible!

THE DAY THE WORLD SLOWED TO A STOP

I would be remiss if I didn't also mention another major occurrence from that same time. On February 1, 2020, the International Committee on Taxonomy of Viruses announced severe acute respiratory syndrome coronavirus 2 (SARS-CoV-2) as the official name of a new global virus. This name was chosen because the virus was genetically related to the coronavirus responsible for the SARS outbreak of 2003. While related, the two viruses were different.

The World Health Organization announced COVID-19 as the name of this new virus, following guidelines previously developed with the World Organisation for Animal Health and the Food and Agriculture Organization of the United Nations.

COVID-19, short for coronavirus disease 2019, became a term that was burned into the psyches of everybody who had access to media and the internet, and well beyond. The ensuing panic that resulted, warranted or not, caused everything to shut down almost overnight. Everyone from federal to local governments and municipalities told restaurants and bars, music festivals and concerts, and all public gatherings, including churches and gyms, to shut their doors. South by Southwest, one of the biggest music and media interactive events known in Austin, was told to cancel. Austinites and music fans around the world were shocked at such an announcement. This had been one of the largest moneymakers for Austin, if not the largest. Soon after, all public gathering places and most businesses were told to close, and people were instructed to shelter in place. The plan was to shelter the healthy and the sick and shut down America. This had never been done before. Even during the Spanish flu of 1918, which was much deadlier than COVID-19, we only sheltered the sick and vulnerable, not the healthy and strong as well. For how long? Nobody knew. It seemed that life as we knew it in the free world was no longer truly free—we were being held hostage in our own homes by this virus, or by the governments who wanted to keep us from overrunning hospitals in what was soon to be known as "flattening the curve."

As it turned out, COVID-19 was here to stay for years to come. I needed to find a way to not only remain strong throughout the pandemic but to actually become stronger, to restart, realign, and grow my transformation and bodybuilding in a new light. The added benefit to this restart was that statistically, the healthier I became, the less likely I was to catch COVID-19. We all needed to remain strong and healthy if we expected to overcome this pandemic.

SCOTT'S GYM POST-COVID

March 16, 2020, was the day that changed my approach on how to rehab, continue to gain strength, and move forward with the transformation I had begun nine years back. This was the day Austin, Texas, started to lock down everything due to COVID-19.

In the weeks that followed, I made a strategic and tactical decision to not only start weight-bearing training but also to ramp up my regimen. I had recently found a trainer (Brian) and a brand-new support staff (Ed, Garrett, and Brad) to come alongside me in my transformation. However, I now had to do this outside of a traditional gym or workout facility. Because of my former physical therapy with Brad, I had been utilizing rubber bands to strengthen my left shoulder while building my right shoulder and arm at the same time (on my own).

With the pandemic now an additional force to be reckoned with, it was time to go all in, at least as it applied to my gym workouts. I officially opened "Scott's Physical Therapy Gym" in my home, or rather, mostly in my garage, knowing that we were about to slide into an even worse predicament—total shutdown, lockout, and isolation. Instead of doing what most people were told to do, which resulted in becoming afraid of being anywhere near other people, I welcomed the sunlight and fresh air. Gold's Gym, my nationally run local gym, had locked its doors literally overnight after I had worked out there just the night before, and other places of fitness training were being severely pressured to do the same. Brian had been furloughed at Crunch Fitness when they were told to shut down, and he was now considered unemployed, alongside all the other trainers.

I asked Brian if he wanted to make a couple extra bucks on the side by meeting me either at "my gym" or at his place to continue our training. He was not only thrilled that I would trust him to continue my rehab during these times of uncertainty, but also, I provided an opportunity for him to keep generating income. At the same time, Garrett and Ed at NeuFit were still allowed to see patients on a one-on-one basis, since PT was still deemed an "essential service" for the time being.

On March 25, 2020, Governor Abbott ordered a shelter in place order for Austin, Texas, and on July 2, Texas Executive Order GA-29 was set in place regarding the proper use of face coverings; moreover, no one was allowed to travel or meet for nonessential business. It was still unclear whether working out outside was permitted, but all other forms of public social commerce came to an abrupt halt. I decided to buck the system and continue working out outside with my new team due to my doctor's orders.

My plan was set. Brian and I met two times a week at my place or his for strength and endurance PT, and Ed and I worked three times a week at NeuFit for physical therapy on both my left and right side. I would also drive twenty miles or so up into Cedar Park, Texas, to work out at Flex Fit, a small family-operated gym that remained open, for my resistance training.

FILLING A NEED

I met Jason Pineda, the owner and operator of Flex Fit rehab and training studio in Cedar Park, through a series of encounters when I was given a guest pass at his gym to work out with Lonnie before the COVID lockdown really took effect. Lonnie and I go way back. We had worked together in the semiconductor field at Applied Materials in Santa Clara, California, where I was an engineer technologist. Lonnie would invite me up to Flex Fit, where I was always eager to try out a new place to flex my fitness goals. Jason and I soon formed a friendship as he learned of my transformation story and wanted to join the team in my rehab and continued transformation. Due to COVID-19, which forced other gyms to close their doors, I would meet him at Flex Fit to work on max loading and other techniques I could not do at home or with Brian. Jason was able to keep his facility open because he offered rehab services that were still listed as *essential* services at that time. He was very generous in allowing me and my team to continue my therapy rehab in order to maintain my set targets.

For the rest of my workout regimen, when not with Brian or at Flex Fit, I worked out at my home gym with my bands and functional equipment. As the weeks went by, I added inventory to my workout collection. I purchased a TRX band suspension system along with a simple sissy-squat rig (for legwork), a set of five-, eight-, and twelve-pound body bars, an abdominal rollout wheel, a pull-up bar, and a set of flat and tube-style bands of varying resistance, along with a stability ball and my favorite: a pro version of the BOSU ball. Most of this equipment I had already been using inside the gym, but now that traditional gym access was no longer an option, I decided to take this added financial hit and go for the gold.

The BOSU ball is fantastic for core and stabilization work. Combined with body bars and resistance bands, I was able to start stability and body work, including muscle sculpting and fine muscle control, especially on my CP side. I used TRX and the rubber bands to strengthen upper- and lower-body muscle groups using my own body weight as well as dynamic band loading. I used the pull-up bar and Versa Gripps wrist straps to stretch out my right and left arms by simple hanging. Then, adding flat bands attached to the bar and around my feet, I began the slow and painful process of relearning how to do a simple pull-up. Both my weak CP right arm and my left shoulder and arm had to work together to lift my 185-pound body off the floor (my post-multi-surgery weight).

On the cardio and endurance side of the gym, I amped it up as well. I began to use a training mask, a technique that Garrett had shared with me (which is now included in his book) that simulates high altitudes up to 18,000 feet by restricting the air intake and exhalation.[80] Then I added a series of weighted workout vests and weight carriers. I came up with this idea from my time up in Gunnison at Colorado Fitness. Even though I could not return to Gunnison at this time to train on the mountain or in a gym at altitude, couldn't I bring Gunnison high-altitude workouts to Austin and increase my output?

I began to use both the training mask and a twelve-pound vest for running and a twenty-pound vest with the training mask to hike, run, and do other cardio work. Both techniques rapidly increased my stamina, lung capacity, and heart health and were excellent in strengthening and reinforcing proper diaphragmatic breathing techniques. A surprising added benefit was that my resting heart rate decreased by thirty-three points during my transformation, and I no longer became tired during long periods of extended exercise activity. By the time we were required to wear masks out in public, like going to the grocery store or working out in corporate gyms once they reopened, I would wear my training mask for the full effect, which also served as a novel solution to our Texas GA-29 face-covering order.[81] Upon reading the finer details within this order, I soon realized that contrary to popular public perception, you did not actually have to wear a face covering while working out. This was due to the potential for buildup of carbon dioxide that could lead to passing out (hypercapnia). This was an omitted fact that most major corporate gyms neglected to share within their own mask requirement orders. Hypercapnia is not a problem with my training mask, as this mask is designed to expel carbon dioxide without the possibility for buildup.

While wearing my training mask, friends soon commented that I looked like Bane from *Batman* and sounded like Darth Vader from *Star Wars*. For added effect, I would wear my "Train or Die" hoodie with the mask and my headphones. Folks said I looked intimidating. They said I looked like a Bane-gangster-Vader bodybuilder posed for a serious beat-down workout. I thought it was a nice touch. Novelty apparently took on a little style.

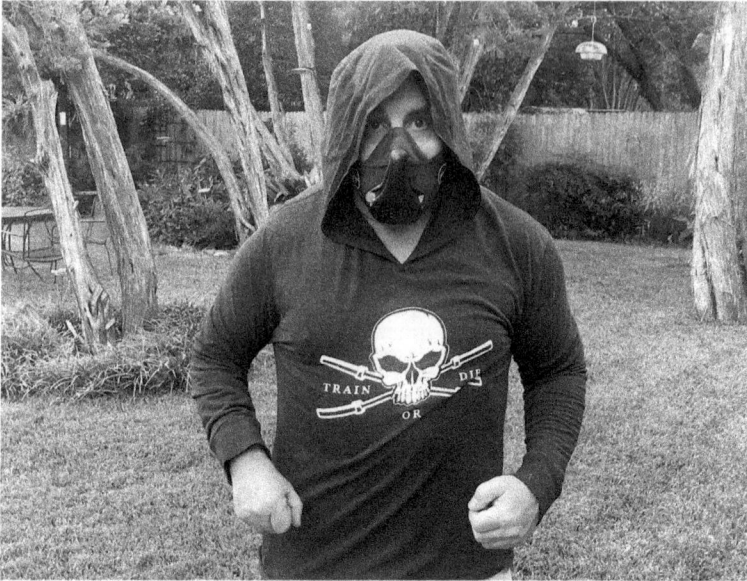

Train or Die hoodie with my Bane training mask

As part of my transformation, I partnered with Garmin in collecting vital workout data for both analysis and fine-tuning my performance. All my workouts were logged using a Garmin Forerunner 935 triathlon watch and triathlon heart rate chest strap (upgraded later to the Garmin Descent G1 dive watch and the Garmin HRM-Pro chest strap) to make sure I stayed within my set limits. I recorded workout data, including calorie burn at every stage in the online program I had created years ago for this project. All calories in and all calories out were recorded along with all my workout data and vitals.

As I mentioned previously, the brain loves novelty, and it learns best in novel ways. By conditioning my body as a serious athlete "in training" with these tools and techniques, I was able to build my body back up faster than I was ever able to do in a traditional gym pre-COVID days. I concentrated on building new neuroplastic networks and focused on balance and fine motor–muscular interactions, physique, and sculpting with the added amps of the Neubie at NeuFit.

The plan was now set, and Mighty Mouse was beginning to run faster in a whole new maze.

DYNAMIC TRAINING

The BOSU Balance Trainer, commonly called a BOSU ball, was invented in 1999 by David Weck. It is basically an inflated half-dome pressurized rubber hemisphere attached to a flat, rigid base. BOSU is short for bionic oscillatory stabilization unit. It looks like a blue stability ball cut in half. I have been told that David, the inventor, likes to think of the ball's acronym as standing for "both sides utilized."

I have traditionally used the BOSU for core, balance, and stability training with my various trainers. However, I have recently amped up my time with the BOSU by incorporating weight lifting and resistance training into the mix. When the dome side faces up, the BOSU ball provides a squishy, unstable surface while the device itself remains stable. This combination of varying stability allows for a wide range of core and balance work and is great for ankle strengthening. In this position, the BOSU can also be used for athletic drills and aerobic activities. I used this side in the beginning for ankle stability work such as step-ups and timed drills where I would have to fast-twitch step-up then reverse-step. When the BOSU is flipped over so that the platform faces up, this is an "advanced position," and the device is highly unstable, like a 3D seesaw, and can be used for other forms of exercise, such as balance and core strengthening exercises, on an unstable flat base. This is the side I now do most of my resistance and weight lifting work on.

All in all, the BOSU is great at building up core strength and priming the body to be more stable on the ground, hence leading to more stable power under load. I have found that overtraining the body to perform under these stressed, unstable conditions will result in enhanced performance while on solid, firm foundations.

I've found that the BOSU ball turned flat-side up was both the most challenging and the most fun (novel) part of my new workouts.[82] I've been doing this for years now, along with weight lifting tasks and catching medicine balls. I am at the point now where I stand on the BOSU in a heel-to-toe, tight-rope pattern, as opposed to standing with feet shoulder-width apart. This increases the ability to focus on balance while also performing lifting tasks such as body bar presses, cable/band rows, dead lifts, RDLs, and torso turns. I have even integrated bouncing my lacrosse ball into this routine for focusing and for a "reset" when needed. Then, when I add in my high-altitude training mask set at an altitude of 18,000 feet for diaphragmatic breathing control, wham! What a workout!

Using this hypoxic training mask is not only challenging but also quite fun. It serves as a novel way of building new neural networks while keeping my mind preoccupied with proper deep breathing and allows me to recover faster for my next rep or workout cycle. These techniques have helped to lower my heart rate and blood pressure, relax my muscles (muscle tone), decrease stress, increase energy levels, and improve my sleep cycles over time. Conversely, when I do not use the mask and instead "chest breathe" or shallow breathe, this leads to activation of my sympathetic nervous system, or the fight-or-flight response. This is the body's stress response. It raises blood pressure and heart rate, increases muscle tension and respiration rate, increases stress, and decreases energy and mental clarity, all of which you do not want for endurance or weight training.

As a side note, when your body is at a high state of stress for long periods of time, your immune system becomes inefficient. As time progresses, the buildup of minor, trivial irritations can lead to significant issues like anxiety and depression and even frequent illness and infections, all of which I do not want in my workouts or in my life in general.

Of course, this intense workout program did not happen overnight. It has taken me years to master and continues to be a never-ending learning process. However, I have noticed that the more I learn to do, the more I am able to accelerate my ability to accomplish things.

At NeuFit, Ed, my physical therapist, also integrated the BOSU as well as body bars and bands along with the Neubie system. Workouts consisted of a forty-five-minute session with four channels of DC Neubie electricity pulsating at various intensities and frequencies across various muscle and neural groups. The goal was to stimulate and build new neuromuscular memory. Ed's techniques have helped to build new pathways and relieve the pain and inefficient neural signaling within my body that had been getting in the way of my progress.

Novelty is a key component in every one of our sessions. I would go home to Scott's Gym and practice these newly learned muscular skills to "reinforce-wire" into my newly formed muscle map.

By mid-May, I had formed a solid regimen of working out at home for about two hours a day, or with Brian and Ed for an hour or so, plus eating exceptionally clean with a low-carb diet…and recording everything during my transformation. How and what we eat—our diet—tends to make up around 85 percent of any weight-loss program and enables a physical training regimen to be successful. Eating clean, with high protein, low carbs, and healthy fats provides the fuel our bodies need for mental, neural, and physical success. By this time in my transformation and ongoing rehab, people started to take notice of my muscle mass increase and fat percentage drop, along with the novel approaches I employed in my various gyms. It wasn't hard for people to notice my fat loss, from 26.9 percent body fat (129.2 pounds of lean body mass) in February to 15 percent body fat (143.4 pounds of lean body mass) by July. Since most people were trending in the opposite direction during the COVID lockdown, my progress was especially noticeable. I was slimming down and starting to believe that I was getting close to my pre-reckoning physique once again.

I also started experimenting with techniques like intermittent fasting, which both Brian and Garrett recommended. Garrett writes, "The most common intermittent fasting strategy is known as 16:8. With this approach, people consume all of their meals for the day over an eight-hour period and fast for sixteen hours. Typically, this involves eating dinner around seven or eight in the evening and waiting until eleven or noon the following day to eat again."[83] I refrained from any alcohol consumption during this time frame as well. After two weeks on this 16:8 plan, I did not notice any weight change at all. Puzzled at the lack of results, I slightly modified my eating timeframe. My theory was that I was eating dinner too late and too soon before going to bed. I found that if I aligned my eating pattern even more closely with my circadian rhythm, I would be able to lose unwanted weight, recover faster, and have more restful sleep patterns while still gaining muscle mass from working out. I found that modifying my fasting window to start at four in the afternoon, skipping dinner, and not eating again until eight in the morning the next day worked like a charm. This solved my resistance to losing weight in the form of fat. The only drawback I found with this eating window was that eating dinner with other folks became a bit of a problem.

By this point in my transformation, several people who had kids with CP or had CP themselves asked how they, too, could benefit from what they saw in me and this transformation. Of note, some of these people were from other countries. I even received several requests from bodybuilders and those I never thought would look to me for inspiration. Inside my head, I guess I still thought of myself as that shy, introverted kid with CP.

But then something extraordinary happened. With help from NeuFit's newly developed methods and protocols, I began to consciously bend my right toes, something that had not been possible before. The ability to bend my right toes meant that the neural path from my brain to my toes was not only intact but could be activated or taught to fire correctly to achieve better balance and fine motor control of the right side of my body. This proved that there were no limits to my potential because my toes are the farthest point on my body from my brain. If I could work my toes, I could strengthen any and all of my neural pathways.

By June 1, 2020, Brian had amped up my workouts one more notch. He introduced me to the stability ball. I am no stranger to the stability ball, but this introduction was a bit more "froggy," as Brian put it. I would learn how to balance on my knees on this big, round ball. That's right: no feet on the floor, everything on that ball. Ironically, the hardest part of balancing on a stability ball was actually getting onto it. Two and a half weeks later and a lot of core ESTIM work at NeuFit with Ed, and I had mastered mounting and balancing on that stability ball on my knees and even added lifting weights to the mix. Unilateral weight lifting and core twisting were the new norm for me. It now seemed that the BOSU was so old school—I do still use it to warm up for the stability ball, though. I added weighted core turns and body bar hand-to-hand flies as well as single kettlebell delt raises, all in an effort to strengthen my core by moving my center of gravity while on that ball. Brian said the next phase would be for me to *stand* on the stability ball. Really? Wow!

I have come to love the final lines in the song "Another in the Fire." It says that: "I'll count the joy come every battle / 'Cause I know that's where You'll be."[84]

For in every reckoning comes great joy.

PEEPING IT UP

Up to this point in my transformation, I found that most training masks, like the one I had been using, work on the principle of restricting breathing, training your body to work with less oxygen so that you perform better when you have more oxygen. My original thought was that by increasing inhalation effort, I would strengthen my diaphragm, and more red blood cells would be manufactured to carry oxygen to my muscles. This worked…as long as I continued to use the mask for training. But when I stopped using the mask after training or for a sport activity itself, within a relatively short time, my red blood cell count would return to a prehypoxic state known as equilibrium. The only two benefits that seemed to last were efficiency in deep sympathetic breathing and a stronger diaphragm. In the long run, the added energy investment of using the diaphragm and training mask during my workouts paid off, with far greater oxygen absorption, which translates into higher energy levels and better nervous system function.[85]

As I continued to develop this hypothesis, I started to research a medical principle called PEEP and how I could adopt it into my transformation. PEEP is defined as positive end-expiratory pressure, which is positive pressure above atmospheric that remains in the pulmonary airways following exhalation. In simple terms, PEEP allows the athlete to breathe out with a slight positive pressure that slightly slows down the exhalation cycle, allowing more oxygen to be absorbed into the bloodstream and more carbon dioxide to be expelled. Since I had been on a ventilator during three surgeries within a relatively short period of time in 2019, I began researching how these ventilator devices really worked and how our bodies utilize oxygen at positive pressure, a holdover from my mixed-gas scuba diving days, perhaps. My research led me to a new concept that ultimately turned my peak performance training methodology completely upside down.

When I met Dr. Sean Boutros, the coinventor of a unique wearable PEEP device that had just been released, we discussed PEEP in detail. I was fascinated to learn how this adaptation of medical life-support technology had been designed to help athletes perform better by use of a simple wearable device. During our multiple conversations, Sean shared with me a published white paper that went into great detail on how his positive end-expiratory pressure valve has been tested with athletes from sea level to Base Camp at Mount Everest.[86] I was amazed to learn how his device has been proven to improve exercise performance.[87] He calls this unique PEEP wearable device the GO^2.

As it turns out, the GO^2 is nearly the exact opposite of my training mask. It actually increases blood oxygen levels by using the physiological principle of PEEP in a lightweight wearable device similar to a mouthpiece used in scuba diving. This device is similar to the "Relaxator" that Garrett uses at NeuFit.[88] With the GO^2 device, the athlete's inhalation is completely natural, with only a slight resistance on exhalation, which is the principle behind PEEP, and unlike traditional training masks, the GO^2 can be used during training and active competition.

During my various calls with Dr. Boutros, he explained that the GO² device increases performance and is quite simple. He said that any athlete who desires to increase his or her performance can use this technology during almost any training or actual sport. I was impressed with his research and the passion he conveyed during our calls and wanted to experience this PEEP device for myself.

Dr. Boutros went further and provided a fascinating abstract entitled "Wearable Positive End-Expiratory Pressure Valve Improves Exercise Performance," which he coauthored and had published in the *International Journal of Exercise Science* in 2019.[89] It explained the clinical benefits of the GO² device. The analytical engineer in me wanted to know more.

Dr. Boutros describes the GO² device as similar in size to a mouth guard. It applies a positive end-expiratory pressure (PEEP) when the wearer exhales, which in turn opens small air sacs in the lungs that are normally collapsed. By opening these sacs, you can utilize more of your lungs to take in oxygen, therefore improving your overall respiratory dynamics.

I could not wait to try it out for myself. He sent me two: one for aerobic and anaerobic exercise (GO² Performance) and the other for athletes who need a mouth guard (GO² with mouth guard protection). My first cardio workout with the GO² Performance device was incredible. I usually work out for about two hours, with half cardio and half resistance, but my first session with this device lasted more than four hours—I actually had to force myself to stop. If I could hang on for double the training time on my first use, I was eager to spend more time with this technology. It was time to PEEP it up.

Over the next few weeks, I used my GO² whenever I performed resistance training or cardio. I tried it at my various gyms and in the outdoors with my twenty-pound weight vest. I was amazed. The only difficulty I had with using this GO² device was the COVID-19 mask requirements that most of the corporate training facilities imposed on their clientele. Using the GO² device alone was frowned upon at many of the gyms I went to. In these cases, while researching the PEEP device alone, I was not able to wear a mask, so I opted not to patronize these gyms. I wanted to focus on evaluating this technology as intended, without restricting airflow due to any mask. Within just a week, I noticed a real performance improvement. I even took my trusty blood oxygen meter with me to take before-and-after readings during my hour-long cardio sessions, maintaining a heart rate around 145 to 150 beats per minute (75 to 80 percent max heart rate). I was PEEPed for sure. Soon after, I combined the training mask and PEEP device together for an awesome cardiovascular workout experience.[90]

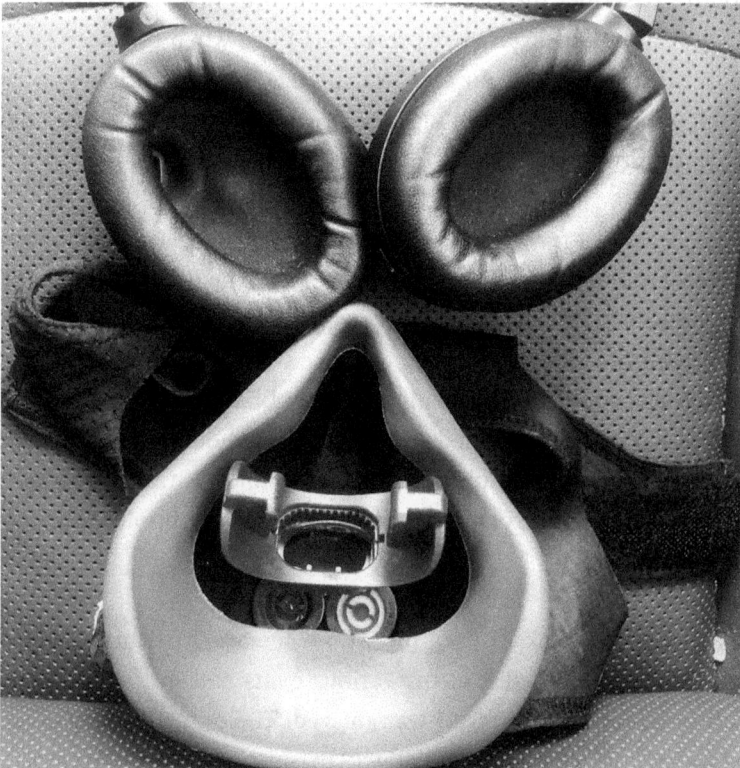

My PEEP and training mask with headphones

THE WORLD STARTS
OPENING UP AGAIN

By the end of May 2020, Texas, along with most of the rest of the United States, started to slowly open back up and allow businesses that did not fold in the great COVID-19 lockdown to reopen. We started to open at a slow 25 percent occupancy rate. On July 2, Texas was once again told to shelter in place and close all bars and social hangouts. Moreover, all persons age six and up had to wear masks while in public per Texas Executive Order GA-29.[91] This lockdown was going to be longer than anyone had ever known before, far surpassing the 1918 Spanish flu outbreak. It looked like the road to opening back up would be much longer than any of us ever thought. It ultimately lasted years. Years that I could not afford to waste.

I was not afraid of social events, but I was concerned about how others reacted to no masks in wide-open outdoor spaces and those wanting to return to the sunlight. We had all been living in a cave for so long that a lot of people were now afraid of public spaces. Crunch Fitness opened its doors again on May 18, and Brian was busy managing the somewhat controlled chaos at his gym. During this time, I reconnected with Jason at Flex Fit in Cedar Park to spend some quality time in his small gym without the hassles of "mandatory" masks and COVID fear running amok. Until the lockdown, Flex Fit had not closed since its grand opening back in 2005. So I was eager to see how Jason's shop was doing. With my twenty-pound weight vest, training mask, and GO^2 device worn under my mask, I went to town on cardio. Headphones cranked up to Hillsong United once more, I was burning calories at high speed, or high enough to get the old heart rate up. I don't know what must have looked scarier…the few people who dared to venture out with cloth and nonsurgical-type masks, or me in the gym looking like Bane in a bulletproof-looking vest and a hoodie that read "Train or Die" in big, bold letters, breathing like Darth Vader doing a 5K run. Or when I was sporting just the GO^2 device, looking like a scuba diver out of water in a hoodie. I did not care; I was once again in the gym. *Train or die.* Yep. That's my motto.

I then increased my weighted cardio sessions by another notch (or three) by switching to a Wolf Tactical plate carrier vest with forty-five pounds and my training mask with PEEP device. Stamina and endurance were mine from this point on.

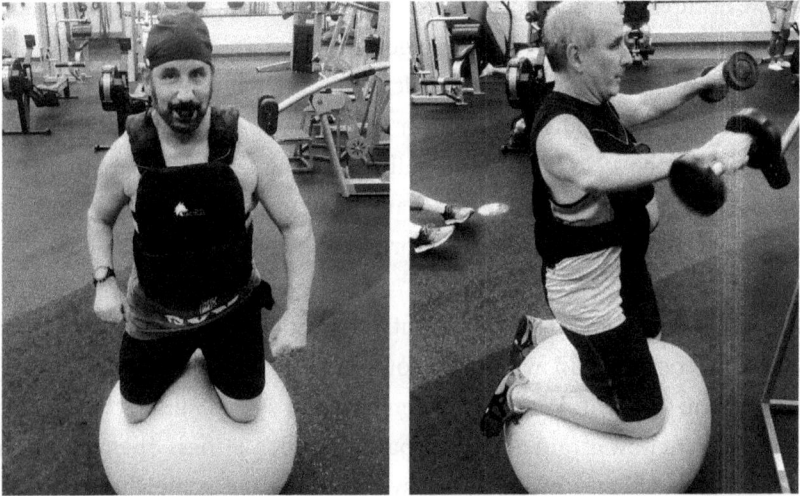

On stability ball with PEEP device and forty-five-pound plate carrier (left) and performing delt raises with plate carrier (right)

The next year was challenging. Both the "social" stigma of being out in public, mask or no mask, and working out in a semi-crowded gym with masks everywhere were daunting to see. Fear of an unseen virus was thick in the air. It seemed that the COVID mask requirements were instilling more fear in people than the virus itself ever could. It seemed that wearing masks subconsciously put people in a constant state of uneasiness. Society was perhaps causing a second wave of panic among the general population. Everywhere you looked, you were reminded of COVID-19. Due to all this paranoia, warranted or not, it became hard to concentrate while working out. Even worse, in the bigger corporate gyms I worked out in, managers were walking the halls, threatening to send the "mask police" in to write people tickets under the premise that "It's for your own health." Was it time to return to Scott's Gym and wait out the storm? I once again bucked the system, trusted God, and remained on course. I started going back to corporate gyms and wore my "Bane" mask with my weighted vest. I had to heal from my injuries and continue forward in my transformation. COVID or no COVID, I was determined to keep moving forward.

TIME TO AMP IT UP

Toward the end of July (2020), I realized I was ready to ratchet it up a notch once more. I would take the plunge and become NeuFit Neubie certified. By this point, I had been working with Garrett's expert staff for over a year, developing and testing protocols for CP. I also decided that with the COVID re-lockdown looming every week, as well as the time and cost associated with my multiple weekly NeuFit PT sessions, I would instead partner with Garrett and purchase my own Neubie system. I would return to Scott's Gym, with occasional road trips for more neuroplasticity gains than if I were to remain on course as it was. This next step in my rehab was both frightening and exciting. It was time to amp it up on my own while still meeting with Brian for strength training once a week and continuing to develop and test protocols for CP with NeuFit.

It was also time to return to Dr. Hall for what I hoped would be my last post-surgical checkup. It had been twelve painful months since the second surgery (one year, two months, and two days from my skydiving accident). Upon my visit, he cleared me to resume more *normal* physical strengthening activity— all but skydiving. Dr. Hall said it would take some more convincing for him to clear me to skydive again due to the accident, lack of ROM without pain, and the level of damage I had endured.

To top that off, I still needed at least eight more months of PT endurance work on my left shoulder if I was ever going to achieve the possibility of full recovery...and he was still unsure of a full recovery. I was so excited to be at this crossroads—except for the skydiving part and more PT. The reckoning had spun me in a completely different direction from just one year ago. The impact and tailspin I sustained in that tunnel turned out to be a course correction that just felt out of control, a major readjustment that set me on a whole new trajectory.

Then, on May 18, 2021, Texas Executive Order GA-36[92] was issued, prohibiting local governments from mandating masks. This signaled to most of Texas that we were done with masking, as the number of COVID-19 infections and deaths were no longer rising and remained flat, if not steadily declining. It felt like the worst might be over and people could start to come out and socialize again.

AN UNEXPECTED SLOWDOWN

Every year since my transformation began, I had been going to my general practitioner for physical exams and blood work to make sure everything was in proper order. And every year, he was amazed at the progress I had made since my last visit. However, during my three surgeries in 2019, my doctor was not as confident that I was on the right path with healing, physical therapy, and strength training. He trusted my new training professionals, but he was concerned that my blood work was not showing the full picture.

During my annual visit in 2019, after surgery number three, my doctor noticed an abnormally low testosterone level in my blood. Not surprising, given that men lose testosterone as we age, but he wanted to keep track of this over the next few months. The next cycle to be tested came before I knew it: my testosterone (TE) levels were even lower, and my energy level was now at rock bottom. By this time (early 2021), I was in rehab five days a week and active in the gym six days a week with my various assigned homework regimens. My doctor wanted to refer me to a urologist to confirm his findings and work on a treatment plan to increase my testosterone. I reluctantly agreed, thinking the worst, and began to research links between low TE and my skydiving accident and three surgeries with extensive rehab—and of course how CP affected all this. As part of my investigation, I researched various treatment options athletes utilize to bring their TE levels back into alignment. Could this work for me, with CP?

I discovered that people with CP tend to expend more energy than able-bodied people—by some reports, as much as 30 percent more energy. This is primarily due to spasticity and other neurological complications around cerebral palsy. The working theory was that this added "energy draw" coupled with the trauma from my skydiving accident and associated surgeries and rehabs most likely caused my body to go into another tailspin. First I hit the *wall*, then rehab, now hormones: another triple whammy.

Two injuries requiring three surgeries in less than a year with extensive rehab, PT, and training would deplete anyone's TE levels. As I learned more about it, I was amazed it had not happened sooner. It seemed that Mighty Mouse had snagged his cape on the corner of a building and was being pulled down once again. My doctor referred me to a specialist who took more blood and performed more tests before recommending supplemental TE shots. It took more than two months of weekly injections and slowing down a little at the gym and in rehab, but it worked. TE pellets were administered shortly after. My insurance company had been reluctant to approve this treatment until physician peer-reviewed consultations took place. It seemed that Mighty Mouse was back to flying once again.

I felt great, and my energy levels on the workout floor had once again returned. The doctors concluded that the abnormal amount of energy that I expend due to my CP and extensive shoulder-injury rehab (along with the overall stress of those three surgeries) had ultimately led to my TE levels dropping dangerously low. If not for my yearly physical exams and a very astute trainer noticing my performance and energy level decline, and blood tests to confirm, I would have hit rock bottom fast without knowing why. I will continue my yearly exams with an added full blood panel workup as time goes on.

SHARING WHAT I HAVE LEARNED:
BRAIN–MUSCLE ALLIANCE

Today, I am no longer that little lion that was late at everything or that simple lab mouse that learned to become mighty and fly. I have once again become an athlete and bodybuilder focused on transforming and sharing this wonderful world of neuroplasticity. My advancements have temporarily slowed down, partly due to the phase of research and recovery I am experiencing, and partly due to lacking an alliance champion (trusted trainer) to push me beyond my own expectations. As my transformation continues and I look towards the future, I am excited to share what I have learned with others, with people who are interested in beginning their own transformational journey.

I often wonder, what if my "older" me could have been there for my "younger" me, to guide and coach younger me through what ultimately took years to learn on my own? My vision is to provide a transformational path—a network of providers, or a referral system of sorts, to connect individuals to professionals in a wide range of disciplines, each of whom could assist with some aspect of their transformation. Doctors, physical therapists, personal trainers, coaches, and other modalities, all networked together to change the lives of others.

As I have shown through my own struggles and triumphs, long-term transformation requires an interdisciplinary approach. I am honored to form such a support system through coaching and encouragement, sharing what works and what does not work, helping others along their journey. This organization of support will form an alliance—between people going through similar experiences, between individuals and providers—with the goal of establishing and improving the body's internal brain–muscle alliance within us all.

I have gone through a lot of physical, emotional, and psychological change and continue to move mountains. What better coach could there be? A coach who keeps reaching up to the skies for that ultimate skydiving adventure yet to come. A coach who will support and teach others and dive deeper into the oceans of transformation. A coach who will provide encouragement, a strong support network through what can be a long and difficult process, and an alliance to help break through the "I cant's" and the "You can't do that's" that we so often believe. This trek is never easy, but it is worth every step.

The Journey Ahead

With Him Nothing Shall Be Impossible

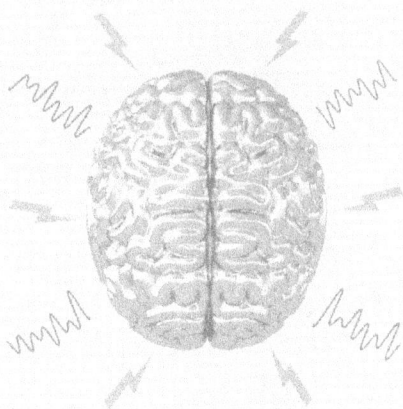

Never Quit
Looking to the Future...

TODAY I FIND MYSELF PONDERING ONCE AGAIN, *How do I raise the bar? Is there even a bar?* This one spirit has endured so much pain, suffering, progress, and vast improvement that my soul has to wonder, can it all be magnified? Can it be replicated? Can I actually help lead others in their own brain–muscle alliance?

I was once paralyzed by my own perception of myself as a small, underdeveloped kid with CP. I falsely believed that I was not worth the effort and could never achieve a sense of "normalcy." Now I know that thinking was an outright lie. It held me back from achieving amazing things. As it turns out, the "experts" were wrong. It turns out I could do what they insisted I could never do—and much more. We should never quit, even when the enemy wants us to. We can all achieve what they say is impossible. We can all do amazing things given the right opportunities, training, and encouragement. As it says in Luke 1:37, "For with God, nothing shall be impossible." We should always be on the lookout for complacency. Complacency can lead us down a road on which we should never travel. In my case, complacency almost took me out altogether (several times, I might add). To that end, I had to endure a life-altering paradigm shift that went way beyond two hours of instruction with a trainer and a gym membership to painfully come to realize this and much, much more.

With many hardships, monumental setbacks, and giant leaps forward in faith, today I am once again an athlete and have resumed bodybuilding. As it turns out, I am, and have always been, motivating and inspiring others to reach way beyond their own understanding and perceived potential—way past their initial preconceived limitations. In a small way, I help motivate others to see the endless possibilities that God wants to reveal in their lives as He has done in mine. I never quite knew how I fit into His plan…until now.

Returning to skydiving is still on my radar. I still have a passion to return to the open sky, but far, far away from walls and bad trainers. Time and continued healing will tell if I will be able to fulfill this dream of mine.

One outcome of this continued journey will include exciting stories of others just like me who have been transformed through their own brain–muscle alliance.

These inspiring examples of folks overcoming struggles and achieving their own goals and dreams (often forgotten or dismissed) will soon be penned and shared to motivate and inspire us all, just as scuba diving or skydiving with cerebral palsy has done (to name a few) in me. I am humbled to be able to come alongside and help lead others through their own personal transformations—leading folks into what God has created them to be.

Until then…

Never let others tell you what your limits are. Cerebral palsy (or anything else) should not keep one from reaching for the impossible because, after all, as it says in Philippians 4:13, we "can do all things through Him" who gives us strength.

Acknowledgments

Robin Cooper—This transformation story and book would never have been possible were it not for Robin, her brother, **Harris Jones**, and her mother, **Bess Harris Jones**.

Bess was the impetus behind the creation of the Austin Cerebral Palsy Center to help Harris and others like me back in 1948. All who grew up in the Central Texas area and had CP in the late 1940s to 1970s were most likely part of the Austin CP Center community. We are all grateful to Bess and Harris.

I give ample thanks to Robin for opening her home and sharing personal memories, scrapbooks, and decades of research, providing this sojourner with a deeper, richer understanding of where I spent the first six and a half years of my life. I have come to understand her family's lifelong passion, which has touched so many kids like me and parents like mine. What an honor it is to include Harris's story within my own life story of triumph over CP. Harris lives on through countless kids today.

Thank you, **Barbara Watt**, for introducing Robin and me.

Kelly and Chris Osness—Kelly, from the very first time I was held outside my immediate family upon adoption into the McCreight family line in 1967, you were there with the caring spirit we all needed. From the early years of endless water-ski tournaments to "babysitting" me as a small tot, we became best friends. When Chris came into your life in Gunnison, Colorado, I rejoiced with you and felt like I had gained a new brother. Thank you both for enriching my life, providing a fertile environment for spiritual growth over these many years, and providing the catalyst for my transformation and this book project. You both offer such deep hope in faith to all who know you, and I know you will have an even bigger impact on countless others to follow.

Lauren Wolf—From the very moment we met in that gym, where you learned of my tattered, crazy story, your kind spirit and deep desire to come alongside my transformation were so incredibly strong. When I was at the lowest point in my rehab (a.k.a. the reckoning), you were determined to put your investigative journalist and deep-dive talents to task in finding out where I came from. From researching DNA records to making countless phone calls, you not only mapped out my entire biological family tree from the very little information I had gathered over the years, but you personally reached out to my long-lost family members for that "first contact" and many that would follow. My once-lost family and I will always be in your debt. It is a joy to count you as a friend.

Lonnie Wendling—My longtime friend. From those early, wild days at Applied Materials, I have known that our friendship would run long and deep. These last few years have been challenging, as well as the most rewarding of my life (so far). You have come alongside me, and through my story, countless others will continue to benefit beyond comprehension. It's such a joy to live life with friends such as you. Thank you for believing in me, for living life together, for helping me through the darkest days of my rehab, for this project, and for our work with BMA. I know the best is yet to come. I look forward to seeing what He has in store for us.

Barbara Munson—Thank you for taking on this project as my first professional editor at Munson Communications. It has been a true joy to have you by my side throughout these last few years. You have taken a vicarious position, learning what it is like to live with CP through my literary work and my transformation story. You gave my story a firm foundation to stand on, correcting my many misspellings and grammar mistakes, and enriching my literary flow along the way. You were able to give my crazy writings a touch of perfection. I could never have done without your expertise of the literary and publishing world. From my first phone call and a high recommendation from John Quinn to the very last edit we worked through, you were always eager to read my writings with such encouragement and grace. Finding a deeper connection in my story through your daughter and son-in-law, Kim and David Anvari, in Gunnison, Colorado, made this book even richer in depth and meaning. I look forward to our next project together.

John Quinn—My good friend John. I have to say thank you for your inspiration over the years. Fate brought us together via common military family experiences and similar struggles with CP, as well as our personal enriching conversations during visits at Miraval in Tucson, Arizona, and in Austin, Texas. I will always cherish eating Texas barbecue and talking about our common foe at the County Line in Austin with you and my family. John, you have always been a fellow sojourner in triumph over CP. Your book, *Someone like Me: An Unlikely Story of Challenge and Triumph over Cerebral Palsy*, has also been a catalyst for bringing my story to press. Thank you for your continued inspiration and support over the years as well as introducing me to Dr. Karen Pape.

Dr. Karen Pape—Although I never had the opportunity to meet Dr. Pape before her passing on June 2, 2018,[93] she laid the foundations and research that ignited my deep desire to achieve more, learn more, and be more than others told me I could be. I had always hoped to meet Dr. Pape and discuss our common drive for kids and adults with CP. I must admit, before I began this project, I did not even know there were different types of CP. I was unaware of the enriching research into this condition made possible by early pioneers such as Dr. Pape. Anyone with the desire to successfully grow stronger with CP really needs to read her book, *The Boy Who Could Run but Not Walk*.[94] Her life's work has been pivotal in the growth of understanding and acceptance in the field of neuroplasticity with regards to CP. She has become a mentor and guide throughout my transformation. My story would not be as rich and deep without Karen's work, dedication, and foundational work with CP.

Eric Kingham—Thank you for keeping me spiritually grounded during the long and tedious days of editing this manuscript prior to and throughout the publishing phase. You persuaded me to stay focused on grace and forgiveness when it seemed, at times, that all I wanted to do (subconsciously) was "nuke it from orbit." Your friendship throughout these many years and a kindred spirit with shoulder injuries, surgeries, and rehab protocols made my pain and recovery bearable—pain tends to bring people together. This book would not have had the spiritual depth it does without your kind and thought-provoking nudges.

Ruth King—God placed you in my life to reshape my paradigm on what amazing, spectacular, awesome possibilities are out there for folks with CP. You kicked my butt. You motivated me, and we developed a friendship that only a few athletes will ever get to fully experience. This is something I will cherish forever. I pray that you will find the way and be a blessing for others like me in years to come.

The workout and PT community—Faith in yourself. One rep is all it takes to start growth. Hope and faith are contagious. Transformation will always follow.

Appendix 1—
Medical Report of Scott's CP

CP Case History—January 15, 1971

Ref. By Dr. Stahr—Fort Worth

Master Scott

Age: 3 1/2

Weight: 29 lb

D.C.: Dr. Stahr

M.D.: Wilburn

      Hudson

Austin Cerebral Palsy Center

PRIMARY SYMPTOMS:

1. Medical diagnosis of Cerebral Palsy

2. Spastic motor contractions of right arm and leg

3. Inability to use right arm and hand at all

4. Possible subluxation of cervical spine

5. Lack of normal speech development for a child of his age

6. Appears to be small in size for a 3 1/2 year-old

CASE HISTORY:

We (parents) first noticed a problem with Scott at five months of age. He didn't reach for toys with his right hand, and he was slow in developing as to sitting up and crawling. He didn't walk until 16 months. His motor development and speech development were slow. He never did use his right hand even with our repeated encouragement. He was taken to a neurologist, who administered an EEG and skull X-ray examination. These were reported to be normal. The doctor felt that there was nothing neurologically he could do for him.

We took him to the Austin Cerebral Palsy Center for an evaluation. They felt that they could help him. He went there five days a week starting at two years of age. He received training in the areas of occupational, physical, and speech therapy.

There have not been any indications of convulsions or seizures. He has been very healthy. There has been no weakness towards respiratory infections. The therapist felt that Master Scott was half a year behind in his motor skills.

Scott seems to be trying to talk more in recent months. He's not very clear vocally. My husband and I can understand some things that he says. He uses syllables and words as opposed to sentences and groups of words. He is saying new words and wants to know the names of everything. He is very inquisitive.

The therapists at the center say that Scott is too young to test for mental ability. They're exercising his arm and he is supposed to wear a weight on his right arm.

Appendix 2—
Medical Report of Scott's Biceps Tear

DR. HALL'S REPORT

Indications for Procedure: Patient presented to Orthopedic Care to my physician's assistant originally on 12/11/2018, and then to me the next day on 12/12/18. At that time, patient had a partial and mild "Popeye" deformity of the left distal biceps, some slight bruising and soft tissue swelling over the distal biceps and upper arm as well as the proximal forearm, and tenderness over the biceps tendon. I performed an ultrasound, which showed at least a high-grade partial-thickness tear if not a full-thickness tear with minimal retraction of the bicep tendon. For verification, I've performed an MRI, which showed a complete rupture of the distal bicep within 2 cm of retraction. Interestingly, the patient actually still had fairly good elbow flexing strength, probably because of his brachialis, and still had reasonable supination strength as well with some minor pain. Because of the complete tear of the biceps and the fact that this is his most functional and strong upper extremity, we decided on surgical repair.

Diagnosis: Left Arm Complete Distal Biceps Tendon Tear.

OPERATION PERFORMED 17 DECEMBER 2018

1. Reinsertion of left ruptured biceps tendon, without tending graph.

2. Incision and drainage, left forearm; deep hematoma.

3. Incision and drainage, left upper arm / elbow area; deep hematoma.

4. *Amnion growth factor allograph injection, left elbow area.*

General anesthetic with the pre-operative nerve block / catheter, Crystalloid and Ancef.

Hardware Utilized: Arthrex Tendon-Side Endobutton with interference screw fixation.

Postoperative Plan: I will keep Scott in a hard cast with soft under dressing for two weeks, and then his elbow brace for at least another 4 weeks after that. No Left Arm use before February 11, 2019. No active range of motion for elbow flexion or forearm supination for a total of 6 weeks, and he may begin starting some light working out (PT) at 3 months post operatively, but no heavy lifting until 9 months postoperatively.

Appendix 3—
Electrical Muscle Stimulation, ESTIM Basics

In the world of ESTIM therapeutic practices, there are three basic electrical waveforms used in commercial electrical stimulation (ESTIM): alternating current (AC), direct current (DC), and pulsed current (either AC or DC in nature). [95]

1. ALTERNATING CURRENT (AC)—KNOWN AS BIPHASIC CURRENT

- Uninterrupted in nature, bidirectional flow of ions; direction changes at least once per second.

- Counted in frequency—the rate at which the current switches direction.

- Electrodes continuously alternate their polarity with each cycle. There is no buildup of charge under the electrodes.

- Two types of modulated AC current used:

- "Russian" current—also known as burst-modulated. Can be either high intensity or low intensity.

  * Interferential or amplitude-modulated.

2. DIRECT CURRENT (DC)—KNOWN AS GALVANIC OR MONOPHASIC CURRENT

- Continuous unidirectional flow of charged particles with a duration of at least one second.

- One electrode is always the anode (+), and one is always the cathode (–) for the entire event.

- There is a buildup of charge since it is moving in one direction, causing a strong chemical effect on the tissue under the electrode.

- Most commonly used with iontophoresis and for wound care.

- Iontophoresis and microcurrent are clinical examples of direct-current interventions.

3. PULSED CURRENT (PULSED BIPHASIC [AC] OR PULSED MONOPHASIC [DC] CURRENT)

- Flow of charged particles stops periodically for less than one second before the next pulse event.

- Pulses can occur individually or in a continuous series.

- Monophasic (DC) pulses do not alternate; pulsed monophasic (travels in one direction only) current allows for a charge to accumulate in biological tissue.

- DC pulsed current utilizes a square wave pulse that "turns on/off" in pulsed fashion and does not alternate or change direction.

Appendix 4—
Medical Report of Scott's Subscapular Tendon Tear

6/7/2019

Dr. Christopher Hall's Report:

Date of Injury: 6/3/2019

Left Shoulder

Location: laterally

Ordered MRI, X-rays, sonograms

> *Scott is here today four days after injuring his left shoulder. He was doing some parachute training at an indoor skydiving tunnel facility under instruction, and hyper-abducted and hyper-extended his left shoulder, and felt a pop in his left shoulder. He has pain in the front portion of it. He also feels numbness and tingling in his left upper*

extremity ulnar 2 fingers. As a reminder, he has cerebral palsy, and this is his unaffected strong left side. He has difficulty reaching behind his back, and some pain with reaching overhead. No previous instability. Also, he has about 5 1/2 months out from his left distal biceps repair, having done great [fully recovered].

His left shoulder has intact skin. He has a little bit of swelling, and minor bruising. He has tremendous difficulty over the bicipital groove, and the subscapular region and lesser tuberosity. He has pain with external rotation, and significant weakness and near inability to internally rotate. Subscapularis lift-off is painful and very weak, indicated subscapularis rupture. He does have range of motion to about 110 degrees, with pain. Negative sulcus sign. He does have some interior apprehension and pain, but no overt instability. He does have pain with resisted use of his supraspinatus against resistance, with slight weakness compared to the other side. He has tenderness over his acromioclavicular joint that does get worse with cross body adduction. He has decreased behind the back range of motion as well. Distal neurologic and vascular status is otherwise intact, other than the slight tingling sensation in his ulnar two fingers.

An MRI, a left shoulder MR arthrogram was performed at Touchstone Medical imaging on June 4, 2019, with the following impression:

1. *Complete tear of the subscapularis tendon with 2.3 cm of retraction to the level of the glenoid.*

2. *Prominent thickening of the anterior band of the interior of the anterior inferior glenohumeral ligament, likely posttraumatic.*

3. *Mild to moderate acromioclavicular joint degenerative change with mild prominent inferior osteophyte.*

4. *Diminutive anterior/inferior labrum*

Upon further inspection, there is a definite slap tear, likely type 2 or 3 present, which is not mentioned in the radiologist report. Also, there is significant tendinosis and at partial-thickness tearing of the supraspinatus tendon, likely high-grade partial-thickness tearing or even areas of full-thickness component of the supraspinatus, again not mentioned above.

I recommend surgery, with examination under anesthetic of the left shoulder to determine any glenohumeral instability, arthroscopic evaluation of the joint with either debridement versus repair versus bicep tenodesis treatment of his slap tear / bicep anchor, evaluation of his labrum and anterior inferior band of the glenohumeral ligament, as well as his rotator cuff, with acromioplasty and distal clavicle excision to assist in decreasing impingement upon his at least high-grade supraspinatus tear (and possible repair of supraspinatus tendon).

He is also interested in regenerative options, such as bone marrow concentrate and platelet rich plasma, to hopefully result in a stronger repair, and possibly lead to an accelerated rate of recovery.

Operation Performed 13th June 2019:

S/P L Subscap repair, bicep tenodesis, claviculectomy, SAD

Successful repair.

Revision Operation Performed 1st August 2019.

Endnotes

1 Gary Schreiber, "45 Miles of Nerves," Be Well World, accessed April 2, 2021, https://www. bewellworld.com/article.cgi?id=Chiropractic_207.

2 Andrew Weil, "Richard Davidson," The 2006 TIME 100, *TIME*, accessed June 17, 2022, http:// content.time.com/time/specials/packages/article/0,28804,1975813_1975844_1976433,00. html.

3 "Cerebral Palsy Myths," LegalFinders, accessed November 7, 2020, https://cerebralpal-sygroup.com/cerebral-palsy/myths/.

4 Called intensive therapy, mentioned in "Programs for Kids with CP Today."

5 For more on speech boards and communication aids, see "Programs for Kids with CP Today."

6 See the chapter titled "College Life for Leo."

7 Jeff Pankin, "Schema Theory" (Massachusetts Institute of Technology, Boston, MA, 2013), http://web.mit.edu/pankin/www/Schema_Theory_and_Concept_Formation.pdf.

8 "Cerebral Palsy Myths."

9 See "The Miami Bust."

10 Amy F. Bailes et al., "Caregiver Knowledge and Preferences for Gross Motor Function Information in Cerebral Palsy," *Developmental Medicine and Child Neurology* 60, no. 12 (December 2018): 1264–1270, https://doi.org/10.1111/dmcn.13994.

11 "Gross Motor Function Classification System," My Cerebral Palsy Child, accessed December 27, 2020, https://www.mycerebralpalsychild.org/diagnosis/gmfcs/.

12 Robert Palisano et al., "Development and Reliability of a System to Classify Gross Motor Function in Children with Cerebral Palsy," *Developmental Medicine and Child Neurology* 39, no. 4 (April 1997): 214–323, https://doi.org/10.1111/j.1469-8749.1997.tb07414.x; "Gross Motor Function Classification System (GMFCS)," Cerebral Palsy Alliance, accessed December 27, 2020, https://cerebralpalsy.org.au/our-research/about-cerebral-palsy/what-is-cerebral-palsy/severity-of-cerebral-palsy/gross-motor-function-classification-system/

13 See "Part 2: Beginnings."

14 *"Her Heart Helps Them to Walk,"* Alcalde, May 1958. Story originally appeared in the March 29, 1953, issue of the *Austin American-Statesman*, written by Mrs. J. Mabel Clark. Minor edits by the *Alcalde* and me.

15 Kate Hunter, "NAPA Centre: How Lynette LaScala Turned Her Son's Near Death into a Two Country, Three Centre Pioneer of Intensive Therapy," Cliniko, August 14, 2019, https://www.cliniko.com/blog/practice-tips/napa-center-pioneer-of-intensive-therapy/.

16 NAPA Website, accessed November 20, 2020, https://napacenter.org/.

17 "Napa Suit Therapy," The Brain Possible, accessed November 27, 2020, https://www.thebrainpossible.com/treatments/napa-suit-therapy.

18 "Intensive Suit Therapy," My Child at CerebralPalsy.org, accessed March 10, 2021, https://www.cerebralpalsy.org/about-cerebral-palsy/treatment/therapy/intensive-suit-therapy.

19 "NeuroSuit," NAPA, accessed November 27, 2020, https://napacenter.org/our-programs/neurosuit/.

20 "First Intensive? 5 Things Your NAPA Team Wants You to Know," NAPA, accessed November 27, 2020, https://napacenter.org/?s=napa+suit.

21 See "Appendix 1—Medical Report of Scott's CP."

22 See "The Gross Motor Function Classification System."

23 Patricia E. Daniels, "The Invention of Velcro," ThoughtCo, updated January 22, 2022, https://www.thoughtco.com/the-invention-of-velcro-4066111.

24 Robert Kraus, *Leo the Late Bloomer* (Young Readers Press, 1971).

25 Karen Pape, *The Boy Who Could Run but Not Walk* (Toronto: Barlow Publishing, 2016), 11–14.

26 Pape, *The Boy Who Could Run*, 122–123.

27 Pape, *The Boy Who Could Run*, 122–123, 192.

28 "SCR Historical Notes," AWSA South Central, accessed July 3, 2022, https://www.awsa-southcentral.com/history/.

29 "What Is the Americans with Disabilities Act (ADA)?" ADA National Network, 2017, https://adata.org/learn-about-ada.

30 "Ski Like No One Is Watching," Ski Teaching Products, accessed March 14, 2021, https://edgiewedgie.com/.

31 See "Part 8: The Reckoning."

32 Pape, *The Boy Who Could Run*, 22.

33 University of Miami SCUBA Club, accessed November 22, 2020, http://www.umscuba.com/.

34 The *Spiegel Grove* was a former US Navy ship and named for the residence of former US president Rutherford B. Hayes.

35 "About MyFitnessPal," myfitnesspal, accessed November 22, 2020, https://www.myfit-nesspal.com/welcome/learn_more.

36 Garrett Salpeter, *The NeuFit Method: Unleash the Power of the Nervous System for Faster Healing and Optimal Performance* (Lioncrest Publishing, 2021), 214–217.

37 Salpeter, *The NeuFit Method*, 218.

38 See training mask and PEEP techniques in "Dynamic Training" and "PEEPing It Up."

39 "Embrace Your Mountain Lifestyle," Treads 'N' Threads, accessed July 3, 2022, https://treadsnthreads.com/.

40 See "Resetting the Bar."

41 Scott McCreight, "Fit Folks," *Austin American-Statesman*, May 19, 2014, https://www.statesman.com/story/lifestyle/2014/05/19/fit-folks-scott-mccreight/10195146007/.

42 David Henning, "An Exploratory Examination of the Role That Lifestyle Activity and Extent of Disability Has on Cognitive Function and Quality of Life in Adults with Cerebral Palsy" (PhD dissertation, Michigan State University, 2020); Lindsay Knof-ski, "A Story of Hope, Courage, Determination, and the Power of God: One Man's Journey

of Rising above His Cerebral Palsy Label to Live His Life to the Fullest" Issues in Diversity, Baylor University, Waco, TX, (paper submitted April 14, 2019), pdf file.

43 Pape, *The Boy Who Could Run*, 279.

44 Melissa Menzez and F. Buck Willis, "Dynamic Splinting for Paediatric Contracture Reduction of the Upper Limb" *Hand Therapy* 16, no. 4 (November 24, 2011): 107–110, https://doi.org/10.1258%2Fht.2011.011019.

45 "Reducing Contractures after Traumatic Brain Injury," *American Occupational Therapy Association: OT Practice* (October 18, 2004): 11–15.

46 Multiple web sources, including "Causes of Lee's Death," BruceFans.com, accessed July 12, 2022, https://brucefans.weebly.com/causes-of-lees-death.html.

47 Pape, *The Boy Who Could Run*, 11–14.

48 Pape, *The Boy Who Could Run*, 19.

49 See "Appendix 2—Medical Report of Scott's Biceps Tear."

50 "Scott Reaches the Impossible with Both Arms," DOC, May 16, 2019, https://www.directorthocare.com/scott-reaches-the-impossible-with-both-arms/.

51 Scott McCreight, "No More Limitations for Man with Cerebral Palsy," *Austin American-Statesman*, May 19, 2014.

52 Chris Davenport and Joel Houston, "Another in the Fire," Hillsong United, 2018, https://hillsong.com/lyrics/another-in-the-fire/.

53 See "Scott Falls from a Plane."

54 See "Appendix 4—Medical Report of Scott's Subscapular Tendon Tear."

55 PT started after my forearm biceps surgery (#1) and shoulder surgery (#2), then had to begin again after revision surgery (#3).

56 Norman Doidge, *The Brain That Changes Itself* (New York: Penguin Life, 2007), 46–47, 50–68, 148–149, 225–226, 239, 275–276.

57 Doidge, *The Brain That Changes Itself*, 48–49.

58 Jim McCambridge, John Witton, and Diana R. Elbourne, "Systematic Review of the Hawthorne Effect: New Concepts Are Needed to Study Research Participation Effects," *Journal*

of Clinical Epidemiology 67, no. 3 (March 2014): 267–277, https://doi.org/10.1016%2Fj.jclinepi.2013.08.015.

59 Sermon notes from Austin Oaks Church, Pastor Brandon Zieske, 2020.

60 Donald Hebb, *The Organization of Behavior: A Neuropsychological Theory* (John Wiley & Sons, 1952).

61 Pape, *The Boy Who Could Run*, 168–169, 286.

62 Three weeks in a similar sling after biceps surgery number one, seven weeks after my first shoulder surgery, and another eighteen weeks post–second surgery, a total of twenty-eight weeks or 196 days.

63 See "One Step Back, Three Steps Forward."

64 DonJoy, *IceMan CLEAR³, IceMan CLASSIC & IceMan CLASSIC³ Cold Therapy Units: Instructions for Use*, 2019, https://www.djoglobal.com/sites/default/files/13-4446-9_B_IFU%2C%20DONJOY%20ICEMAN.pdf.

65 Halo Neuroscience, "The Athlete's Guide to the Brain: Hyperplasticity," *Halo Neuroscience* (blog), February 25, 2016, https://blog.haloneuro.com/the-athlete-s-guide-to-the-brain-hyperplasticity-3686a46f02e8.

66 Pape, *The Boy Who Could Run*, 95–114.

67 Pape, *The Boy Who Could Run*, 104.

68 Pape, *The Boy Who Could Run*, 104.

69 Pape, *The Boy Who Could Run*, 107.

70 Pape, *The Boy Who Could Run*, 130.

71 Pape, *The Boy Who Could Run*, 100–107, 130.

72 See "Appendix 3—Electrical Muscle Stimulation, ESTIM Basics."

73 Salpeter, *The NeuFit Method*, 29.

74 Pape, *The Boy Who Could Run*, 24.

75 Salpeter, *The NeuFit Method*, 29–31.

76 Salpeter, *The NeuFit Method*, 220.

77 Salpeter, *The NeuFit Method*, 215.

78 Refer to the sections "Don't Forget to Breathe" and "Dynamic Training."

79 See "Train or Die—Survival of the Fittest."

80 Salpeter, *The NeuFit Method*, 217.

81 Governor of the State of Texas, Executive Order GA-29 Relating to the Use of Face Coverings during the COVID-19 Disaster, Austin, Texas, July 2, 2020, https://gov.texas.gov/uploads/files/press/EO-GA-29-use-of-face-coverings-during-COVID-19-IMAGE-07-02-2020.pdf.

82 Interesting aside: the BOSU ball actually has a disclaimer to not use it with the flat side up! It says, "standing on platform not recommended."

83 Salpeter, *The NeuFit Method*, 233–234.

84 See also Romans 5:3, James 1:2.

85 Salpeter, *The NeuFit Method*, 214–215.

86 Bradley S. Lambert, *Go2 Results Report* (Houston: Houston Methodist Orthopedics & Sports Medicine), accessed December 26, 2020, https://cdn.shopify.com/s/files/1/0065/8253/4197/files/Test_2_-_GO2_vs._Nothing_Test_Results.pdf?1747.

87 Stephen F. Crouse et al., "Wearable Positive End-Expiratory Pressure Valve Improves Exercise Performance," *Sports Medicine and Health Science* 2, no. 3 (September 2020): 159–165, https://doi.org/10.1016/j.smhs.2020.06.002.

88 Salpeter, *The NeuFit Method*, 217.

89 Alexandra L. Remy et al., "Wearable Positive End-Expiratory Pressure Valve Improves Exercise Performance (Abstract)," *International Journal of Exercise Science* 2, no. 12 (2020), https://digitalcommons.wku.edu/ijesab/vol2/iss12/62/.

90 See "The World Starts Opening Up Again."

91 Governor of Texas, Executive Order GA-29.

92 Greg Abbott, "Governor Abbott Issues Executive Order 36 Prohibiting Government Entities from Mandating Masks," Office of the Texas Governor, May 18, 2021, https://gov.texas.gov/news/post/governor-abbott-issues-executive-order-36-prohibiting-government-entities-from-mandating-masks.

93   Karen Pape, accessed December 25, 2021, https://karenpapemd.com/.

94   Pape, *The Boy Who Could Run.*

95   Christina Howard, "Three Major Types of Current Used in Electrical Stimulation (estim)," (lecture, Lane Community College, Eugene, OR, 2019), https://media.lanecc.edu/users/howardc/PTA101/101FoundationsofEstim/101FoundationsofEstim4.html.